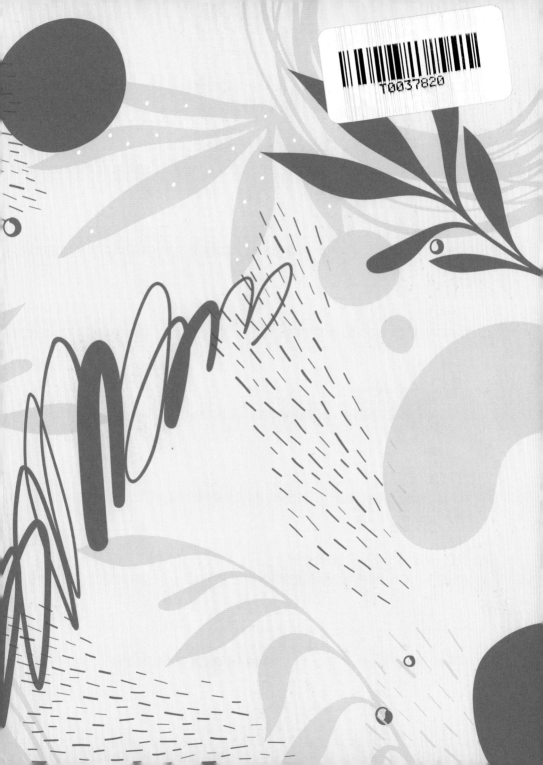

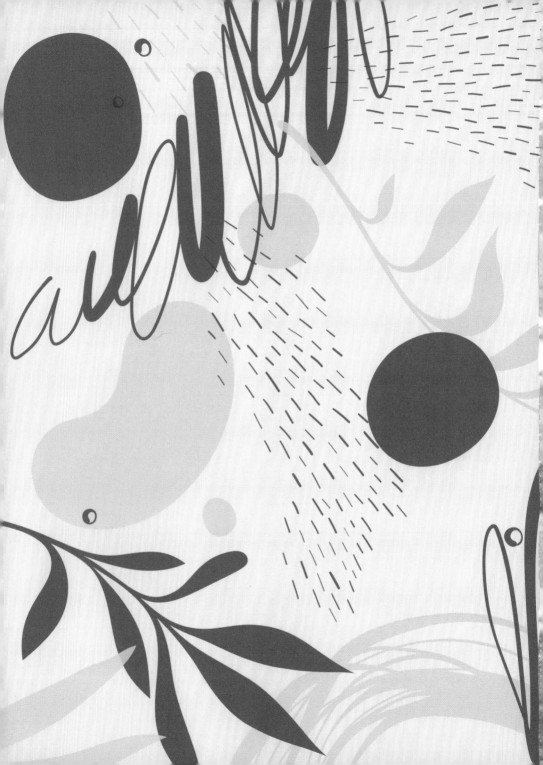

The
Clean Living
Handbook

The
Clean Living
Handbook

80+ All-Natural Soaps, Cleaners,
Detergents & Nontoxic
Household Products

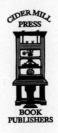

CIDER MILL
PRESS

BOOK
PUBLISHERS

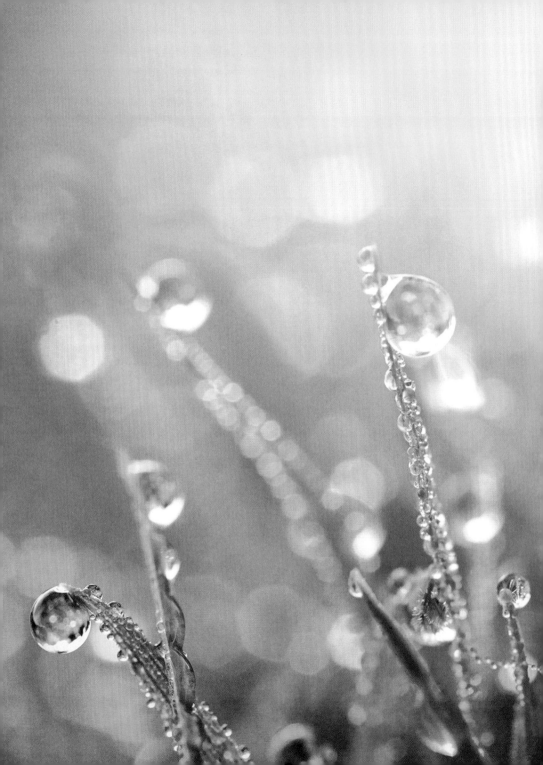

CONTENTS

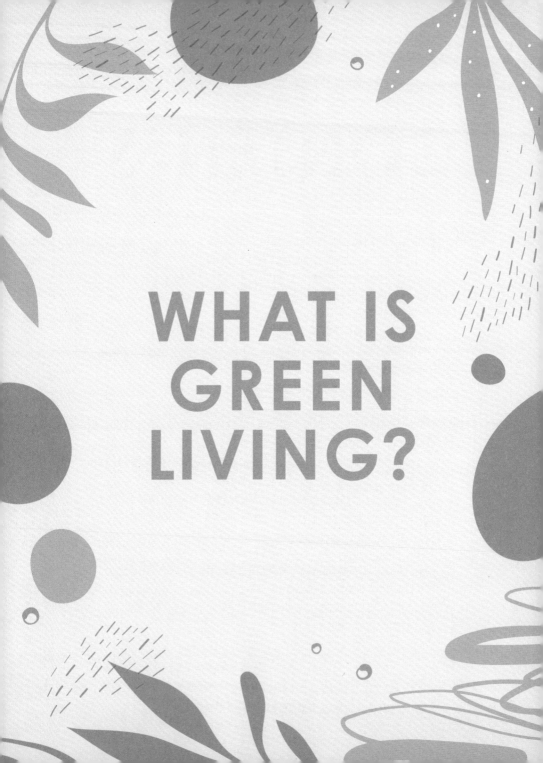

WHAT IS GREEN LIVING?

For many of us, our concern for the well-being of the planet, as well as our health and quality of life, coincides with milestones of our own independence—renting our first apartment, buying our own home, and raising our children. Well into the 21st century, it's difficult to ignore the connection between our daily life choices, large or small, and their environmental and health impacts. The products that we use to clean our living spaces and our bodies constitute one of those daily choices that can make a big difference, not only in how we treat the planet, but also ourselves.

The lab-created chemicals and petrochemicals that we've embraced since World War I and the Atomic Age are coming under increasing scrutiny for their health repercussions. From disposable cleaning pads to plastic spray bottles with unrecyclable parts, the single-use plastics feel exceptionally wasteful in a time where the outcomes of human-driven climate change are inescapable.

Green living means acknowledging that we are not separate from the environments in which we live. Our bodies—minds included—are made of an assemblage of organic materials constantly in conversation with the air we breathe, the water we drink, the land from which we get our food, the materials we use for clothing and shelter, and a million

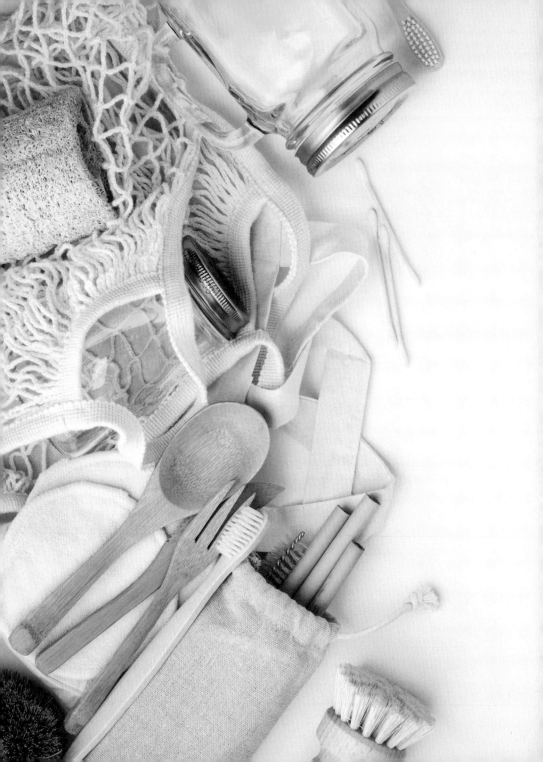

other things. Green living means taking all that into account in order to make those relationships better on both sides—for us and for the environment.

If that's important to you, and you are ready to make some changes in your daily habits to get there, then this book is for you. And if you feel a responsibility toward the planet—not only for yourself and your family, but for future generations as well—then read on. As Jonas Salk, the inventor of the polio vaccine, once said, "Our greatest responsibility is to be good ancestors." The most crucial part of being a good ancestor is being a good steward. That means standing up for yourself against the pressures to consume and pollute.

THE RISE OF CHEMICAL PRODUCTS

When and why did we abandon traditional, clean, homemade cleaning products and transition to store-bought, complex chemical products? In short, just over 100 years ago, advances in chemistry and technology affected all walks of life. These advances coincided with "the gospel of germs," when the war against tuberculosis, Spanish flu, and other pandemic diseases caused by microbes was fought with any weapon available. Between 1909 and 1929, American per-capita spending on cleaning supplies and chemicals increased by a factor of seven. But the fever to use chemicals caused some to try to resolve previously settled problems. For example, did you know that early dry cleaners used raw gasoline?

Unfortunately, the science behind making industrial chemicals has always been way ahead of the regulation of the side effects or unforeseen consequences of the regular use of these chemicals—and that continues to this day.

1889: Lysol antiseptic is introduced in Germany, containing a poison called cresols. Throughout the early to mid-20th century, Lysol is used by some as an underground abortion method.

1931: Procter & Gamble develops Dreft, the first synthetic laundry detergent in America, based on formulas the company had found in German chemical plants in the wake of WWI.

1953: A survey of American pediatricians finds that poisonings make up half of the accidents they treat in children.

1960: The Federal Hazardous Substances Labeling Act requires any dangerous household product to be vividly labeled as such. "Keep out of reach of children" label language becomes ubiquitous.

1977: A family of a toddler whose esophagus dissolved after drinking a small amount of Liquid-Plumr (she was treated and survived) wins a $500,000 out-of-court settlement from the Clorox Company.

2020: Johnson & Johnson discontinues its talc-based Johnson's Baby Powder product. However, the company, facing a lawsuit from 38,000 people claiming the product contained asbestos, says that it's not because the product is dangerous, but rather that people aren't buying it because of "misinformation."

2021: A lab finds very high levels of benzene, a carcinogen, in two antiperspirant products made by Procter & Gamble, sparking a series of lawsuits that are yet to be resolved.

2022: A CDC study finds glyphosate—a toxic farm chemical in widespread use since 1996—in 80 percent of urine samples.

2022: Taking 19 samples of fresh snow from across a large area of Antarctica, scientists discover microplastics in 100 percent of the samples.

2022: A *Chicago Tribune* investigation uncovers that 8 million Illinois residents are potentially drinking PFAS—forever chemicals made by chemical companies—in their tap water.

It's hardly any wonder that a 2022 Gallup poll found that 41 percent of Americans had "very little" or no confidence in big business—and the numbers were worse still for the criminal justice system, which routinely allows polluters and companies whose lawyers help them run out the clock to escape accountability. More than ever, it's important to watch out for yourself and your loved ones.

THE MOVE TO GREEN LIVING & ZERO WASTE

"Zero Waste" as defined by the U.S. Environmental Protection Agency (EPA) is a moving target. Among the many definitions put into writing by organized groups ranging from the United States Conference of Mayors to the City of Pasadena, certain common themes emerge. At the top of the list is this: we can—and should—put fewer things in landfills and, in general, use up fewer of Earth's resources.

If you have a Zero Waste goal, try asking yourself these types of questions:

Do I need this cheap shirt from the mall?
Or can I go to the thrift store and give new life to
an already-made article of clothing?

Do I need to drive my car to the big-box
store to get this ingredient for tonight's meal?
Or can I walk to a neighbor's house and see if they have it,
thereby strengthening the social bonds in my community
while refusing to burn fossil fuel?

Do I need to buy this jug, bottle, or box of
commercial cleaning product? Or can I make my
own from natural ingredients, thus saving on packaging
and energy costs and preventing mystery chemicals from
entering my home and the environment?

Recycling, composting, reusing, and declining to use in the first place are the steps that people like you take toward the goal of Zero Waste. It may seem impossible—setting out a bag or two of trash per week is nothing unusual—but maybe you can think of one small step that can get you on your way.

INDOOR AIR QUALITY

Among the categories of indoor air pollution listed by the EPA, one of the easiest to exercise any level of control over is "products for household cleaning and maintenance, personal care, or hobbies." There's little you can do about industrial air pollution in your area, or what pesticides your neighbors use, or even what types of ovens, furniture, or building materials are in your house. But by choosing clean living products, you can make your home a cleaner environment. Taking control of your most intimate microclimates—your kitchen, your bathroom, the common areas of your home, and your yard—can be accomplished with simple steps and under a manageable budget.

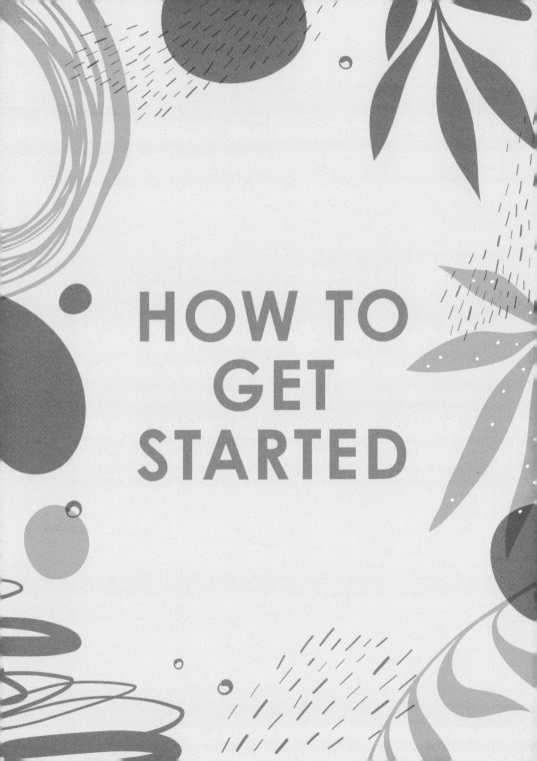

HOW TO GET STARTED

First, take stock of what you already have. Look in your kitchen for the basic building blocks of your green-living, Zero Waste inventory. Start with tools and materials: glass jars, spray bottles, stainless steel and glass pots, and wooden and silicone stirring spoons. Then look in your linen drawers and closets for natural fibers: cheesecloths, tea towels, microfiber cloths, and natural sponges. If you plan on making your own soap, do you already have a kitchen scale, immersion blender, and slow cooker? If you plan on making your own kombucha or fermenting your own vinegar, do you already have large glass containers?

From there, look for the Big 6 ingredients: vinegars, oils, abrasives, essential oils, soaps, and water. What do you already have? Setting up a solid foundation of sustainable, renewable versions of these ingredients will help you put together a green-living, Zero Waste household.

THE BIG 6

The substances here are the real heroes of the green-living home. If you have them already, great. If not, plan to accumulate them over time as you begin your journey.

VINEGARS

When yeast—single-celled fungal organisms—eats the sugars and starches in the juice from almost any plant, the liquid ferments into an alcohol solution. That's the first step in making vinegar. Next, over a fermentation period ranging from a couple of weeks to many months, the alcohol interacts with oxygen and acetic acid bacteria. These bacteria consume the alcohols left by the yeast, producing acetic acid in the process. That's all vinegar is: a solution of acetic acid in water (vinegars typically have a pH of around 2.5). Vinegars contain 4 to 8 percent acetic acid (4 percent is the minimum acidity required to prevent the vinegar from spoiling).

DISTILLED WHITE VINEGAR

White vinegar is made from alcohol from fermented grains (barley or corn, usually) that has been purified by distillation. Unlike other vinegars, it has little flavor since it's basically pure acetic acid and water.

APPLE CIDER VINEGAR

Apple cider vinegar, or ACV, is made from fermented apple juice. Rich in antioxidants and probiotic bacteria, it has been used as medicine for thousands of years.

CASTILE SOAP

Castile used to refer to a soap whose fat content was supplied by olive oil and which was made in the Castile olive-producing region of Spain. Today, it simply means a soap made from the oils of plants.

Until recently, the way most Americans encountered castile soap was in the form of the eye-catching blue, purple, orange, green, and other colorful labels of Dr. Bronner's Pure-Castile Liquid Soap, spotted on the shelf in a neighborhood health food co-op. But lately, castile soap has taken on cultural significance as the kind of soap that has only natural, plant-based ingredients—nothing synthetic or petroleum based—and is easy on the skin, extremely versatile, and pleasantly scented. You can buy liquid castile soap at most supermarkets. See pages 41, 42, and 49 for recipes to make your own.

According to the American Cleaning Institute (ACI), archeologists date the first use of soap back to ancient Babylon in 2800 BC. However, even after the discovery of soap, the ancient Mesopotamians, Greeks, and Romans were still bathing using only water, then dousing themselves in fragrant oils. After allowing the oils to soak in, the ancient Romans used a scraping tool to scrape off the oil.

Aside from the ancient Syrian city of Aleppo—home to possibly the world's oldest soap bar industry—soaps had a consistency somewhere between the bars and liquid castile soaps we know today: goopy and used primarily to clean fabrics. In fact, American pioneers still looked at soap as just a way to clean clothes and sheets. It wasn't until the 19th century, when new factories took the business of saponifying animal fats and lye to scale, that using soap to clean skin and hair took off among the masses.

DISTILLED WATER

Distilling regular water removes impurities and minerals. When the water is boiled and the steam collected, it leaves the heavier substances dissolved within it behind—which, in the case of your metal pipes, leads to limescale problems (see page 84). Minerals are what gives regular water its taste. Since distilled water contains no minerals, it is completely tasteless. In this book, distilled water is used as a pure carrier for other ingredients.

ABRASIVES & EXFOLIANTS

Some recipes in this book call for alternative abrasives: sugars, coffee grounds (both used and fresh), and salts. Abrasives grind away at buildup, whether it's burnt food in your oven, sebum on your skin, or grease on your countertops.

BAKING SODA

Baking soda is a powdery, white substance that is safe to use in a wide variety of ways. When heated to 400°F, baking soda—sodium bicarbonate ($NaHCO_3$)—breaks down into three substances: carbon dioxide gas (CO_2), water vapor (H_2O), and washing soda, or sodium carbonate (Na_2CO_3).

WASHING SODA

Washing soda is a common eco-friendly product that you can usually buy off the shelf at your local supermarket. However, if you want to be sure that you're not using something with additives, you can easily make your own. Many recipes in this book call for washing soda. Just remember that washing soda is not the same as baking soda: with a pH of 11, washing soda is more caustic than baking soda, which has a pH of 8.1. You should wear rubber gloves when handling washing soda. Use washing soda in cleaning situations where you want something natural but powerful.

CARRIER OILS

Carrier oils, made from the nuts of trees by cold-press processing, serve to dilute and "carry" essential oils. They don't evaporate like essential oils do, and they have a fairly neutral taste and aroma, albeit distinct for each oil—the difference between olive oil and avocado oil is easy to notice. Each contributes its own blend of vitamins, beneficial fatty acids, and moisturizing properties. Here are the carrier oils called for in the book:

JOJOBA

Jojoba oil comes from a desert shrub (*Simmondsia chinensis*) native to Mexico and the American Southwest. It is nongreasy and therefore great for skin applications. It's rarer and more expensive than most other carrier oils.

GRAPESEED

Grapeseed oil comes from the seeds discarded by the wine-making industry. It's thick, neutral smelling, and very moisturizing, and therefore excellent for massage-related uses.

OLIVE

Olive oil has been used for thousands of years in the Mediterranean, for everything from cooking to bathing. Extra-virgin olive oil is very minimally processed and therefore is richest in antioxidants and vitamins.

AVOCADO

Avocado oil is pressed from the pulpy flesh of avocados (*Persea americana*). Clear and colorless, it has a very high smoke point, so it's great in cooking. It's rich in beneficial fatty acids and has a thick consistency, making it a good choice in complex skin- and hair-care products.

SWEET ALMOND

Sweet almond oil is pressed from the pits of varieties of the almond tree (*Prunus amygdalus*). This oil has a yellowish tint and a light, nutty scent. It's amazing on skin.

ROSE HIP

Rose hip oil comes from the pressed roots of roses. This clear oil has a neutral aroma and good dermatological properties, and is best used in recipes that call for serious moisturizing.

ESSENTIAL OILS

Essential oils are volatile, and they evaporate quickly. Because they were cold-pressed from citrus fruit rinds or collected from the steam distillation of plant stems, leaves, or flowers, they pack a lot of aroma power. Essential oils should not be eaten and they usually need to be diffused in water or in carrier oils when using them topically.

PRACTICAL MATTERS

Before diving into this book, familiarize yourself with these basic processes that are common in the recipes that follow. Skip ahead if you're already a pro.

HOW TO STERILIZE REUSED GLASSWARE

Place any jars or dropper bottles upside down in a large pot of boiling water for at least 10 minutes. Set out in the sun to air dry completely before using.

DIY DOUBLE BOILER

For recipes calling for gentle heat to melt ingredients such as coconut oil and shea butter together, a double boiler is an easy option. It may be better than using the microwave, which can heat certain areas a lot while leaving others cold.

You'll need a medium pot and a glass or metal mixing bowl. Add water to the pot until it is about one-quarter full, or even less, then bring it to a soft boil or a steady simmer on the stove top. Place your bowl of ingredients in the pot. The bottom of the bowl should be resting above the top of the water or just barely touching it. As the steam heats the bottom of the mixing bowl, stir your ingredients slowly to melt them together.

DO A PATCH TEST BEFORE APPLYING

If you're unfamiliar with a skin-care ingredient, such as a new carrier oil or essential oil, first do a patch test by applying a very small amount of the ingredient to a small area of your skin. Wait awhile. If there's no negative reaction, then you can proceed with your project in confidence. The same goes with some cleaning supplies on certain surfaces. If you're about to clean that heirloom walnut dresser with a new cleaning spray you've just made, test the spray out on a small, discreet area first and wait to see what it does before proceeding.

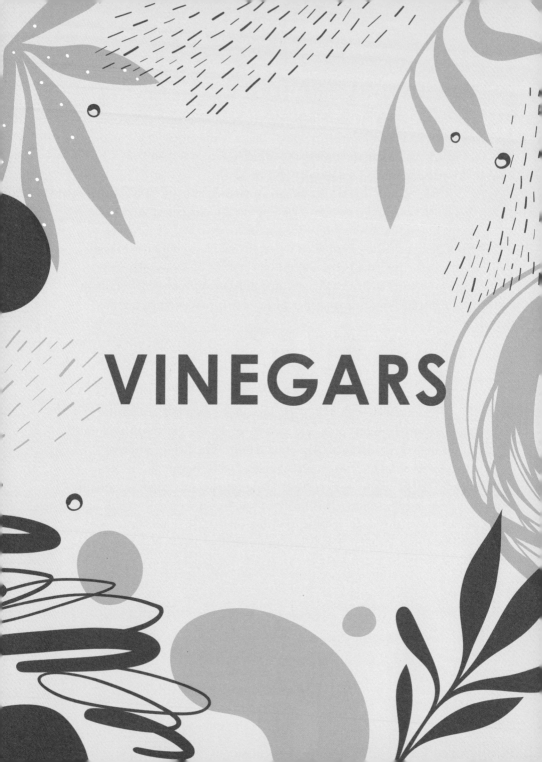

VINEGARS

Many recipes in this book call for vinegar, which is an extremely eco-friendly and healthy ingredient. Making your own vinegar is an increasingly popular green-living practice.

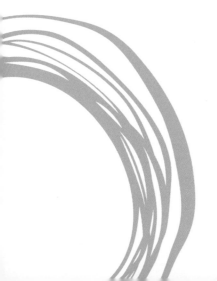

Kombucha Vinegar

If you're already a kombucha maker, this will be easy: simply set aside a batch to ferment for 1 to 2 months instead of the usual 6 days to 2 weeks. If you're not a kombucha maker, read on! One-gallon sun tea jars are large enough to make a decent-sized batch and will work for this recipe.

Ingredients:

1 gallon water

6 to 8 bags black tea

1 cup organic raw sugar

1 to 2 cups unpasteurized kombucha (store bought, from a friend, or reserved from a previous batch)

1 SCOBY, at least ½ inch thick (see sidebar)

1. Using a large stainless steel pot, boil the water, then add the tea bags and sugar. Remove the pot from heat.

2. Cover the pot and allow the tea to cool to room temperature overnight. Leave covered.

3. Once cooled, pour the tea into a large (at least 1 gallon) wide-mouth glass jar or ceramic container for the SCOBY to live in. Don't use plastic.

4. Add the kombucha and gently stir.

5. Add the SCOBY to the jar. It should begin to float to the surface right away, though it is okay if it is submerged—it will get in the right position by itself.

6. Cover with parchment paper, a folded tea towel, or a coffee filter, and attach securely with a rubber band or twine around the mouth of the jar. This will prevent mold and fruit flies from getting into your kombucha while allowing air in.

7. Let it sit for at least 1 month before doing a taste test. Once the taste is suitably "vinegary," it's ready to use. If you want regular kombucha for drinking, you can simply stop the fermentation process earlier.

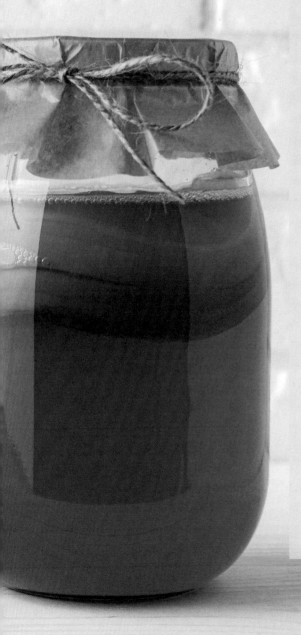

To get into kombucha making, you'll need to acquire a SCOBY—symbiotic culture of bacteria and yeast. This is the flat, alien-looking organism that produces kombucha as a by-product of ingesting the right nutrients, found in the Kombucha Vinegar recipe. If you have a friend who already makes kombucha, ask for a layer of their SCOBY, in at least 1 to 2 cups of their brewed kombucha. Otherwise, simply buy a plain, store-bought kombucha drink and let the bottle sit out—opened but loosely covered—until it forms its own SCOBY.

The first time you make kombucha may take longer, as your SCOBY needs time to grow to the size of the container. The larger your SCOBY, the faster it will make your tea into kombucha.

To prevent mold or bacteria from ruining your SCOBY, always handle the SCOBY with clean hands, only use sanitized containers and implements, and never leave the SCOBY or tea exposed for more than a few minutes at a time.

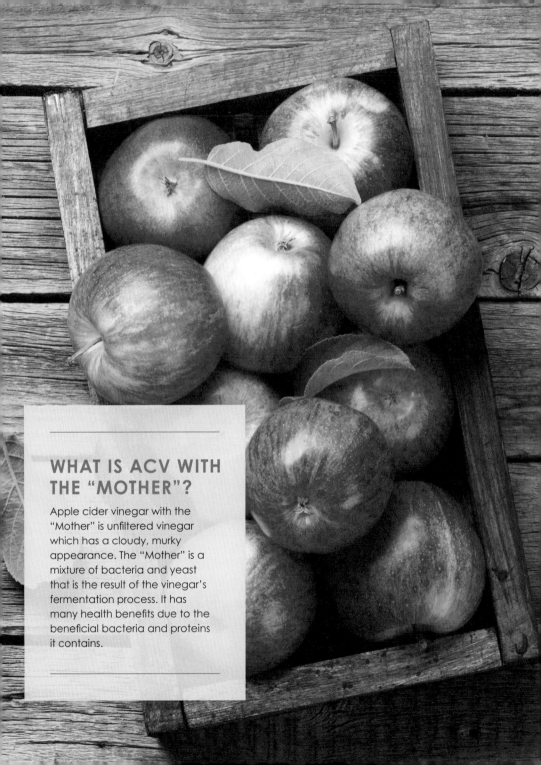

WHAT IS ACV WITH THE "MOTHER"?

Apple cider vinegar with the "Mother" is unfiltered vinegar which has a cloudy, murky appearance. The "Mother" is a mixture of bacteria and yeast that is the result of the vinegar's fermentation process. It has many health benefits due to the beneficial bacteria and proteins it contains.

Apple Scrap Vinegar

Did you know you can reuse your apple scraps—peels, cores, and ends—to make apple cider vinegar? Try out this recipe with some of the cleaning recipes in this book and compare against store-bought apple cider vinegar. If yours works just as well, that's an accomplishment!

Ingredients:

Scraps from 16 organic apples

1 cup organic sugar

1 gallon distilled water

2 tablespoons apple cider vinegar with the "Mother"

1   Cut up your apple scraps into smaller pieces to increase the surface area of the apples and remove any rotten parts.

2   Set the scraps in a sterilized 1-gallon wide-mouth glass jar, then pour the sugar in. Shake together.

3   Add the distilled water and apple cider vinegar. The apples should be fully submerged under the water. Use a fermentation disk weight if you have one.

4   Use a piece of clean cloth or coffee filter and a tight rubber band to cover the mouth of the jar. You want air to be able to get into the jar, but not any bugs. Set the jar in a location where it won't be disturbed.

5   Several times per day for the first 3 to 6 days, remove the cloth cover and give the apples a stir. You don't want to give mold a chance to grow on the exposed apples. Immediately put the cloth cover back on. Once the apples sink, you can stop this process.

6   Add a dash of the apple cider vinegar with the "Mother" when you notice your mixture bubbling. After 2 or 3 weeks have passed, you can strain out the apple chunks if you'd like.

7   After a month, taste the vinegar to see if it is done. If it tastes like apple cider vinegar, then strain the vinegar into sterilized, capped bottles and store at room temperature until ready to use. If not, allow it to continue fermenting for up to 3 months.

Shortcut Apple Cider Vinegar

The success of this recipe comes down to its ingredients. Use good-quality apple juice and get apple cider vinegar with the "Mother."

Ingredients:

3 cups organic 100% apple juice (not from concentrate)

¼ cup apple cider vinegar with the "Mother"

1   In a sterilized, wide-mouth 32 OZ. glass jar, add the apple juice.

2   Give the vinegar a shake and add it to the jar.

3   Place a clean tea towel or other piece of permeable but tightly woven cotton cloth over the jar opening (you don't want fruit flies getting through), pull tight, and secure with a rubber band.

4   Store the jar in a dark location for 2 months, in order for the cultures in the vinegar to work. Check on it weekly, and occasionally taste it to monitor the progress.

5   If the vinegar becomes moldy, discard it and start over. If not, and if it tastes vinegary, transfer it to a clean jar or bottle, straining if desired. Seal it and store it at room temperature until ready to use. If it does not taste like vinegar, allow it to continue fermenting.

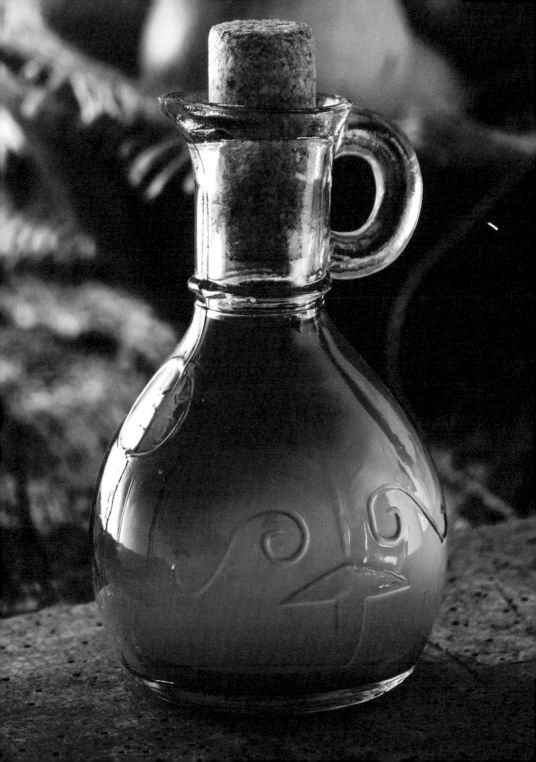

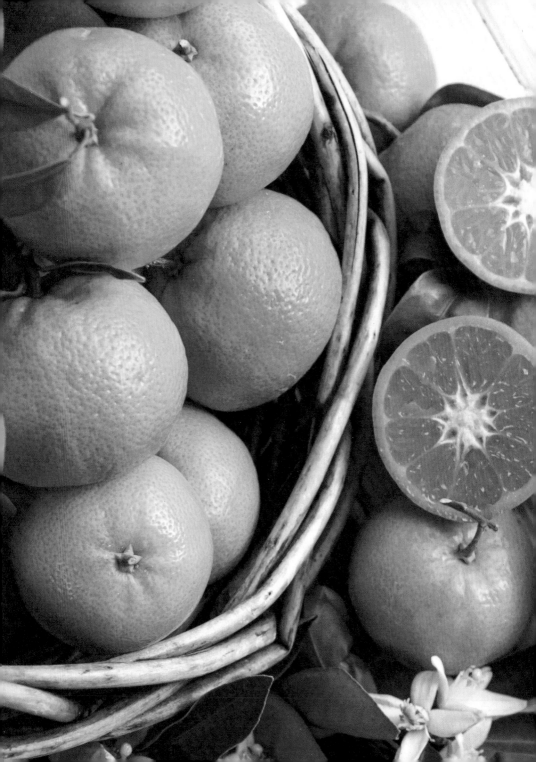

Orange Peel Vinegar

This recipe gives you a way to use those orange peels that would otherwise go into your compost bin. Any recipe that calls for white vinegar can instantly be made more citrusy if you use this Orange Peel Vinegar instead.

Ingredients:

Peels of 2 oranges, sliced into eighths or quarters

1 cup distilled white vinegar

1   Layer the orange peels in a sterilized 8 OZ. glass jar.

2   Pour in the vinegar to fill the jar completely.

3   Set the jar in a dark spot and let it steep for 2 weeks.

4   After 2 weeks, strain the vinegar into a clean 8 OZ. jar.

Banana Peel Vinegar

If your household goes through bananas at a steady clip, or if you tend to have bananas over ripen on your watch, this recipe is your chance to turn that bulky, messy by-product into pure gold. Try adding a splash of this Banana Peel Vinegar to a glass of water, a meal, or any recipe in this book calling for vinegar.

---

1 Wrap the chopped banana peels in a natural cheesecloth and tie closed.

2 In a large pot set on high heat, add the distilled water and bring to a boil.

3 Lower the cheesecloth bag containing the banana peels into the water and boil for 5 minutes.

4 Turn off the heat and allow the pot to cool.

5 Once cool, remove the cheesecloth bag and squeeze it thoroughly to get all of the banana peel juices into the pot. Compost the banana peels.

6 Add the sugar to the pot and stir.

7 Pour the banana-peel-extract-and-sugar solution into one large, sterilized canning jar or several smaller canning jars. In each jar, leave a headspace.

8 Add the yeast and use a cloth and a rubber band or lid ring to seal the jar against bugs. Allow it to ferment for 7 days.

9 Decant or strain the liquid to remove the solids, pouring into a sterilized jar or jars. Add the apple cider vinegar. Cover with the cloth again and allow it to ferment.

10 After 2 weeks, carefully, without contaminating the vinegar or leaving it uncovered for more than a few minutes, test the taste. If it's vinegary, it's just about ready. Allow it to ferment for up to 2 months, testing every so often.

11 When it's ready, boil the vinegar in a large pot for a few minutes to pasteurize. Allow it to cool, then seal in jars until ready to use.

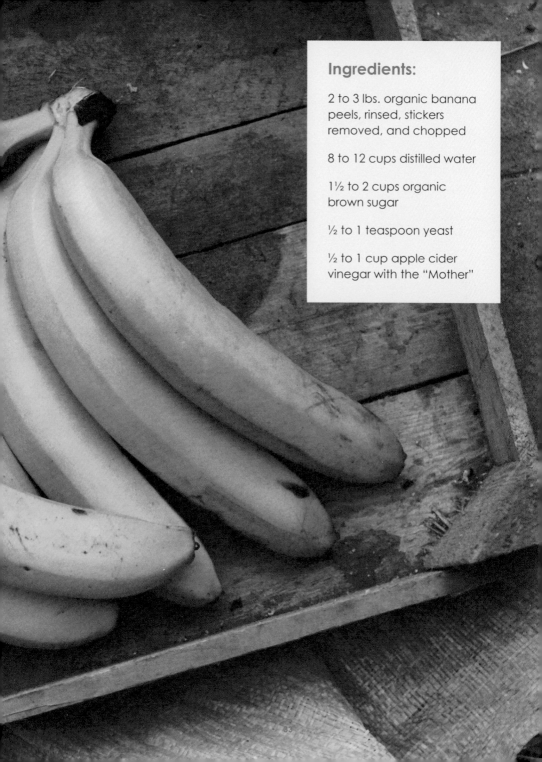

Ingredients:

2 to 3 lbs. organic banana peels, rinsed, stickers removed, and chopped

8 to 12 cups distilled water

1½ to 2 cups organic brown sugar

½ to 1 teaspoon yeast

½ to 1 cup apple cider vinegar with the "Mother"

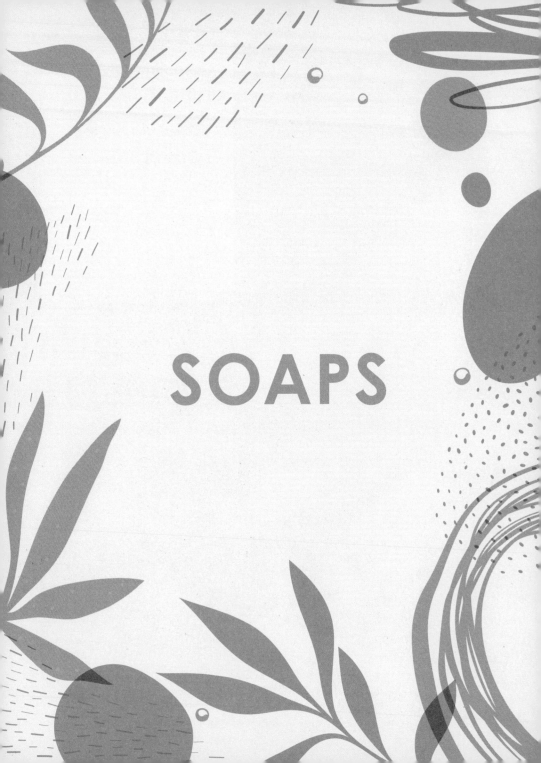

SOAPS

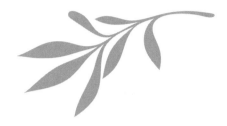

Saponification: the chemical process
of turning lye (alkaline substances) and
oils (fatty substances) into soap.

At the advanced level, one of the staples of true green living and cleanliness is soapmaking. In this section, there are recipes for soap bars and liquid castile soaps. All are customizable, and the liquid castile soaps can be used in many of the recipes in this book. For all soap recipes, use the precise amounts given, especially if you're new to soapmaking. Otherwise, your soaps may be inconsistent or ineffective. To save on labor, have an immersion blender and a large slow cooker ready to use.

Almost any container can become a soap mold: antique wooden boxes, takeout containers, plastic food-storage tubs, plastic shell cases used to protect vegetables, even iPhone boxes or Pringles cans. Often, you'll still have to cut your soap bars down to size after they've cured in their molds—you can buy a soap knife or make do with what you have in the kitchen already. Avoid using metal other than stainless steel for your molds, as any unsaponified lye residue will react with it.

KNOW YOUR LYE

There are two kinds of lye: sodium hydroxide (NaOH), or caustic soda, and potassium hydroxide (KOH), or caustic potash. The more common is sodium hydroxide, which is used to make cold-pressed soap bars. You can buy sodium hydroxide products in big-box stores or supermarkets, but it may be easier to order it online.

It's possible to make potassium hydroxide yourself using rainwater, wood ashes, and patience (see page 38), but it's also available to buy at big-box stores or online. Potassium hydroxide is used in liquid castile soap recipes (see pages 41, 42, and 49).

SOAPMAKING SAFETY

The first and most important thing to know about lye is this: **never pour water into lye**. It will explode. Instead, you must always pour the lye into the water. When you add lye to water, there is a chemical reaction that gives off heat and noxious fumes, so stand back and don't breathe them in.

The second thing to know is that lye is very caustic—with a pH of at least 13—and is dangerous, both in terms of breathing in its by-product gasses and contact with skin or eyes. Therefore, when working with lye, it is critical to be fully awake and aware, to work outside on a pleasant day (or at least in a well-ventilated space), and to wear proper protective equipment (see below). You also need to set up where you can be sure that neither kids nor pets will go and there will be no interruptions. Finally, keep lye stored in a safe place when not in use.

WHAT TO WEAR:

- Goggles that fully cover your eyes (required)
- Rubber gloves that extend up to your elbows (required)
- Rubber or leather apron (recommended)
- A mask (recommended)

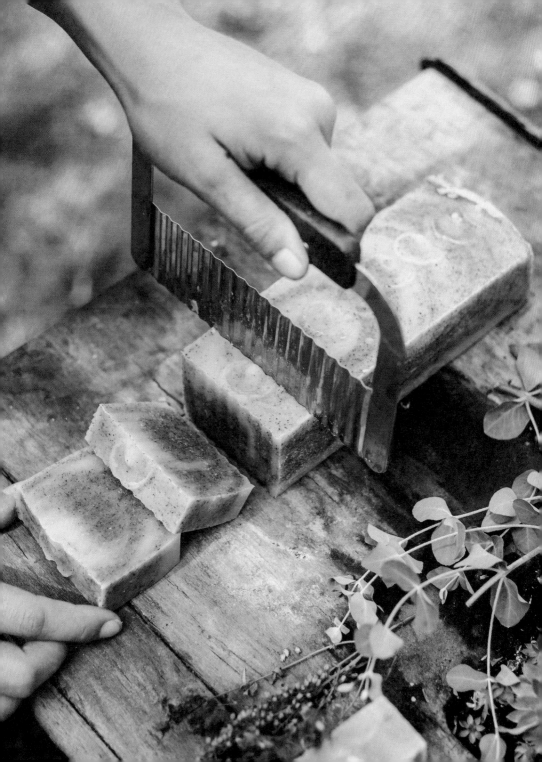

Rustic DIY Potassium Hydroxide (KOH) Lye

This recipe will make you feel like one of the ancient Romans who first discovered the saponification process. According to ancient Roman legend, soap got its name when rainwater from Mount Sapo would wash down the mountain and mix with animal fat and ashes. They realized that the resulting clay mixture made cleaning easier. If you have a firepit that you use regularly, or know someone who does, you're halfway there.

1   When you're planning to make your lye, set out buckets to collect rainwater—beneath your downspouts before a storm is ideal. Additionally, the ashes you're collecting should be stored in a sealed plastic or stainless steel container.

2   Find a large terra-cotta pot with a drainage hole in the bottom. Alternatively, drill a hole or holes in the bottom of a five-gallon bucket or wooden barrel.

3   Cover the bottom of the pot with a layer of pebbles topped by a thick layer of pine needles and/or straw. You can add an intermediary layer of sand if you wish. Your filter layer should be several inches thick.

4   Fill the pot with ashes and tamp them down so they are well compacted. Then, using 2x4s or another stable perch, set up the pot so that it will drain into a large, stainless steel pot for collecting.

5   Tip the rainwater into the pot so that the water comes nearly to the top. Let it sit so the water slowly drains into the collecting pot, overnight if necessary. Whatever water is collected is caustic and should be treated with care.

6   Once you have roughly a gallon of brown- or amber-colored lye water, you need to test its pH level. To do this, GENTLY set a potato in the water. If the lye is the right pH, it should float. If it sinks, you will need to rerun the lye water through the ash pot (avoid splashing). If the potato floats to the top immediately, the lye water is too strong and should be slightly diluted. Remove the potato and discard.

7   Store the lye in a well-labeled plastic or stainless steel (no other kind of metal) container until ready to use in soapmaking.

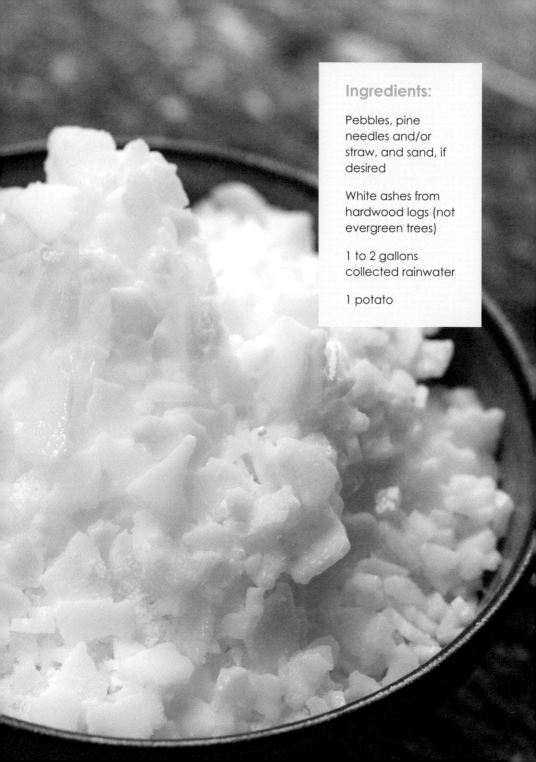

Ingredients:

Pebbles, pine needles and/or straw, and sand, if desired

White ashes from hardwood logs (not evergreen trees)

1 to 2 gallons collected rainwater

1 potato

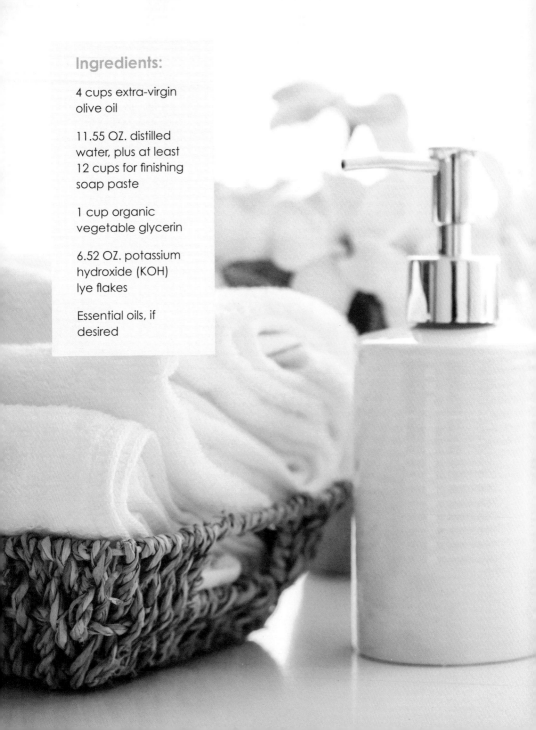

Ingredients:

4 cups extra-virgin olive oil

11.55 OZ. distilled water, plus at least 12 cups for finishing soap paste

1 cup organic vegetable glycerin

6.52 OZ. potassium hydroxide (KOH) lye flakes

Essential oils, if desired

True Liquid Castile Soap

Liquid castile soap—a traditional soap made with olive oil—should be clear. The glycerin accelerates the saponification process while contributing extra moisturizing capability to the finished soap. Note that if you're going to use this soap as a base to add to more complex recipes, you may want to leave it unscented. If you want to use homemade lye solution (see page 38), add the glycerin to it before combining it with the oil in batches, eyeballing the consistency and erring on the side of too little lye. If you don't have glycerin, substitute with the exact same amount of distilled water.

1 Using a large crockpot or slow cooker set to low, heat the olive oil.

2 In a large stainless steel pot, add the distilled water and glycerin, then stir.

3 Working safely (see page 36), add the lye flakes to the water-glycerin mixture. Stir gently until the water clears up.

4 Add the lye-glycerin mixture to the warm olive oil and stir to combine. If you want to scent your liquid castile soap, add a few drops of your preferred essential oils.

5 Use an immersion blender to whip the mixture up into a soap paste. Keep blending until the soap paste is custardy, then cover and slow cook on low heat for 3 to 4 hours, stirring occasionally. If you don't have an immersion blender, use a stainless steel whisk or spoon or a wooden spoon (note that it's a lot more work to do it this way). The soap will reach a thick, translucent gel state.

6 Test the soap. In a jar or bowl, pour ½ cup of distilled water. Add a heaping spoonful of soap paste and stir until dissolved. Wait for a few minutes. If the diluted soap mixture remains clear, you are ready to move to step 7. If it's cloudy or scummy, cook for another hour, then retest.

7 To finish the liquid soap, working in batches, add the soap paste to distilled water (or rainwater) in a ratio of 1 part soap paste to 3 parts water and let rest overnight, stirring occasionally. You can use pots or large glass jars.

8 When the soap is fully liquid, bottle it in your container(s) of choice and store until ready to use.

Olive & Coconut Oil
Liquid Castile Soap

The coconut oil makes this castile soap recipe extra sudsy, making it a nice choice for using as an all-purpose hair and body wash in the shower. Stored in small, squeezable bottles, this all-natural soap is a perfect choice for camping trips. Note: if you want to use homemade potassium hydroxide lye solution (see page 38), add it to the oils in batches, eyeballing the soap paste for consistency and erring on the side of too little lye.

1 Using a large crockpot or slow cooker set to low, melt the coconut oil, then add the olive oil, stirring to combine.

2 In a stainless steel pot or bowl, pour 4 cups of distilled water.

3 Working safely (see page 36), add the lye flakes to the water. Stir gently until the water clears up.

4 Carefully add the lye solution to the oil mixture in the slow cooker and stir to combine. Add a few drops of your preferred essential oils if you would like your soap to have a fragrance.

5 Use an immersion blender set on low to whip the soap paste to a custardy consistency. Stirring occasionally, cover and continue to cook the soap paste on low heat for 3 to 4 hours. The soap will reach a thick, translucent gel state.

6 Test the soap. In a jar or bowl, pour ½ cup of distilled water. Add a heaping spoonful of soap paste and stir until dissolved. Wait for a few minutes. If the diluted soap mixture remains clear, you are ready to move to step 7. If it's cloudy or scummy, cook for another hour, then retest.

7 Add 10 cups of distilled water to the slow cooker, still on low heat, stirring to agitate the soap paste. Leave overnight. If the mixture is still cloudy, add more distilled water.

8 Bottle the soap in your container(s) of choice and store until ready to use.

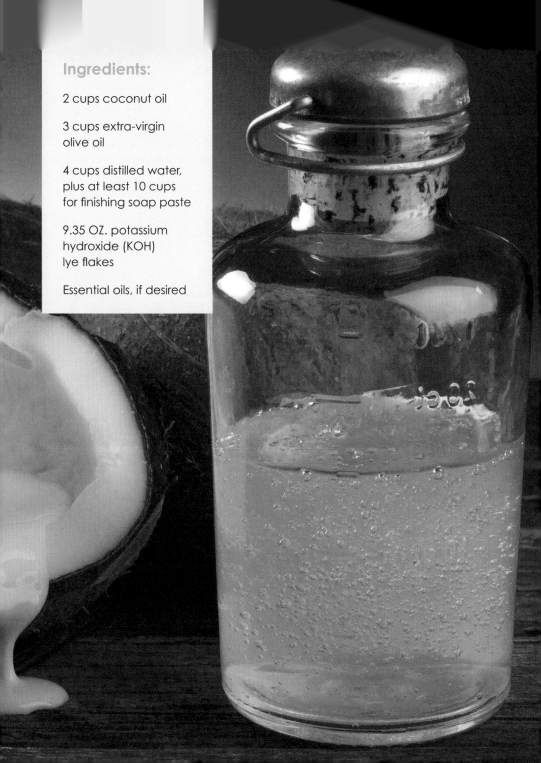

Ingredients:

2 cups coconut oil

3 cups extra-virgin
olive oil

4 cups distilled water,
plus at least 10 cups
for finishing soap paste

9.35 OZ. potassium
hydroxide (KOH)
lye flakes

Essential oils, if desired

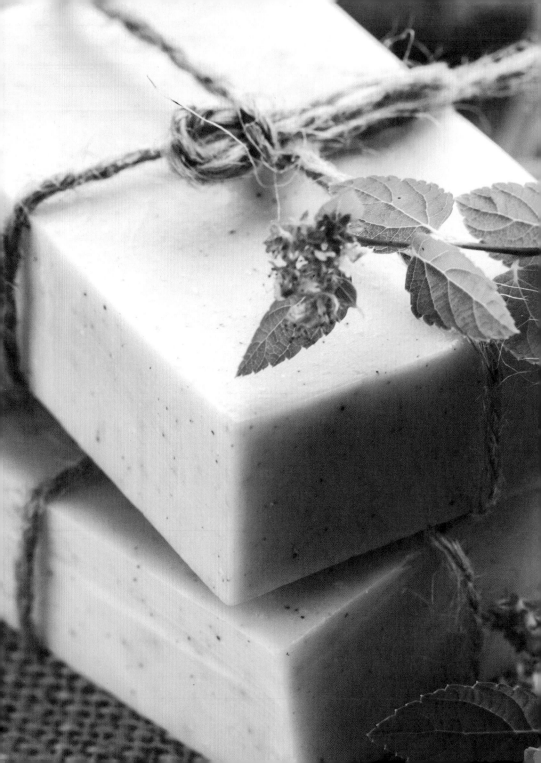

Simple Long-Cure Single-Oil Soap Bars

If you have the patience to wait more than three months for the curing process to play out, you'll be rewarded with beautiful white bars of really basic soap made from coconut oil. Once you've mastered this recipe, you can move on to cold-processed bar soaps that have more complex mixtures of oils and fragrances. This one-oil recipe is meant for beginner soap makers, but if you want to spice things up, consider adding ground oats, lavender flowers and stems, or rosemary petals, along with any essential oil blends you can think of. And have your soap bar molds (see page 35) ready to go! For this recipe, you'll need a digital kitchen scale.

Ingredients:

150 grams distilled water

66 grams sodium hydroxide (NaOH) lye flakes

454 grams organic refined coconut oil

Essential oils, if desired

Exfoliants or herbs, if desired

1   In a stainless steel pot or bowl, pour the distilled water.

2   Working safely (see page 36), add the lye flakes to the water. Stir gently until the water clears up.

3   Over low heat, melt the coconut oil in a large stainless steel or glass pot on the stove top (this will happen quickly). Once the oil is melted, immediately remove the pot from heat. Add a few drops of essential oils, if desired.

4   Being very careful to avoid splashing, gently add the lye solution to the oil. Mix the soap paste together with an immersion blender set on low until the paste reaches a pudding consistency. If you don't have an immersion blender, you can also use a stainless steel or wooden spoon. Add exfoliants or herbs, if desired.

5   Pour the soap paste into your soap molds and let it sit in a cool, dark place for 12 to 48 hours.

6   Remove the soaps from the molds, cut into bars if necessary, and let cure in a dark, dry place for 10 weeks before using.

Coconut-Orange-Coffee Soap Bars

This soap bar recipe is a bit more complex than the Simple Long-Cure Single-Oil Soap Bars (see page 45), but it cures in only a few weeks, and it packs a few surprises. Get ready for an exfoliating, pungent bath-time experience! For this recipe, you'll need a digital kitchen scale.

Ingredients:

195 grams distilled water

80 grams sodium hydroxide (NaOH) lye flakes

500 grams organic extra-virgin olive oil

100 grams organic refined coconut oil

¾ cup French or Italian roast coffee grounds, drip or espresso ground

40 drops sweet orange essential oil

1 Pour the distilled water into a stainless steel pot or bowl.

2 Working safely (see page 36), add the lye flakes to the water. Stir gently until the water clears up. Set aside to cool.

3 Combine the oils in a large stainless steel bowl, glass pot or bowl, or slow cooker.

4 Carefully add the lye solution to the oil mixture. The warm lye solution should melt the coconut oil if it isn't already melted. Stir to combine.

5 Use an immersion blender set to low to mix the soap paste. When the soap paste reaches a pudding consistency, add your coffee grounds and essential oil and mix everything together.

6 Pour the soap into your molds and set aside somewhere dark and dry.

7 After 24 hours, remove the soap from the molds and cut into bars. Set the bars in a cool, dark place to cure. Allow 1 month for the curing process to finish before using or gifting the soaps.

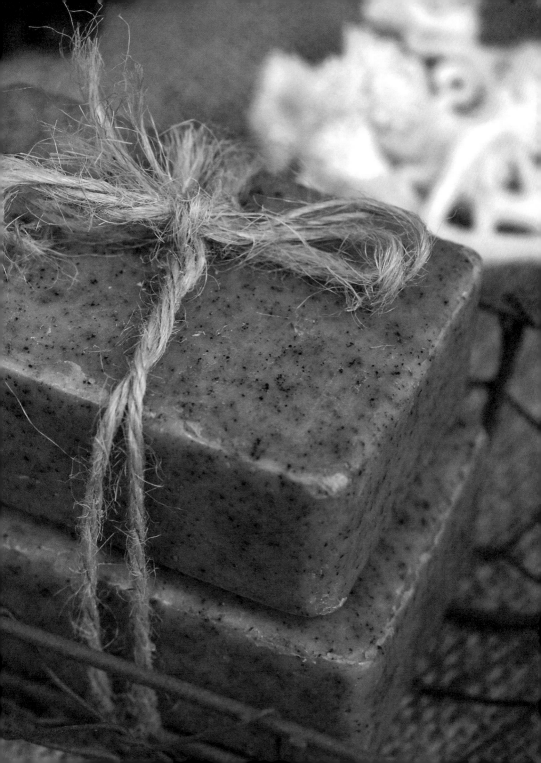

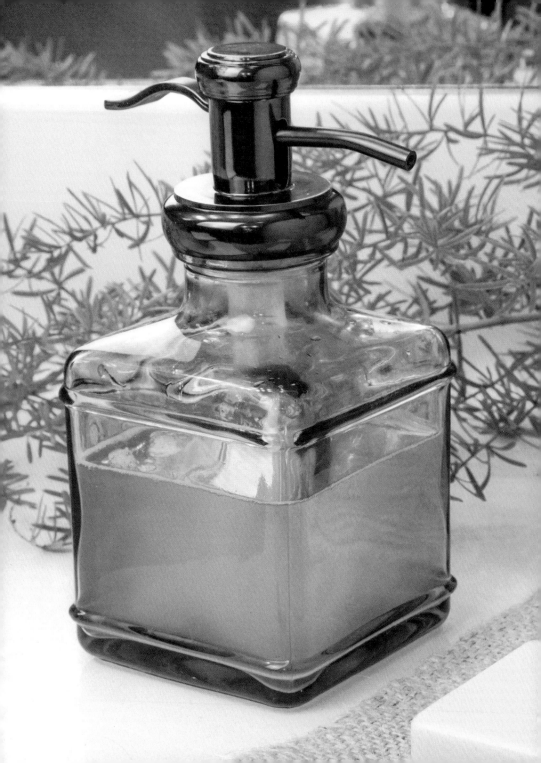

Antibacterial Liquid Castile Hand Soap

Reuse an old hand soap pump for this recipe. Make sure you thoroughly wash it out first. The tea tree essential oil gives this soap an antibacterial oomph. If you're feeling productive, make multiple batches and set out bottles in the kitchen and bathrooms.

Ingredients:

2½ cups distilled water

10 drops tea tree essential oil

2 to 6 tablespoons liquid castile soap or True Liquid Castile Soap (see page 41)

1   Combine all of the ingredients, starting with the distilled water, in your hand soap dispenser.

2   Give it a shake and set out for use. Occasionally, you'll want to shake before using it to reagitate the contents.

NATURAL CLEANERS

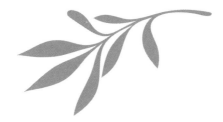

It's time to switch back to the basics. These DIY cleaners and disinfectants are simple and cost-effective. You probably have a lot of these ingredients in your pantry already, and if not, they're very inexpensive compared to cleaning products you'll find on supermarket shelves. As a bonus, you'll drastically reduce your plastic consumption and household pollution caused by the use and disposal of commercial products.

Always label any bottles, jars, or tins of DIY cleaners with all of the ingredients contained inside. That way, you can be sure what each mixture consists of.

Oregano & Tea Tree All-Purpose Cleaning Spray

This recipe is a healthy alternative to off-the-shelf all-purpose cleaners. Reuse or buy a spray bottle. This recipe calls for tea tree and oregano essential oils for their antibacterial and aromatic properties.

Ingredients:

4 cups distilled water

¼ cup liquid castile soap or True Liquid Castile Soap (see page 41)

10 drops tea tree essential oil

10 drops oregano essential oil

1   In a 32 OZ. spray bottle, pour the distilled water and then add the other ingredients.

2   Shake gently to mix, and then shake again before each use.

3   Spray onto the surface you intend to clean, then wipe with a microfiber cloth.

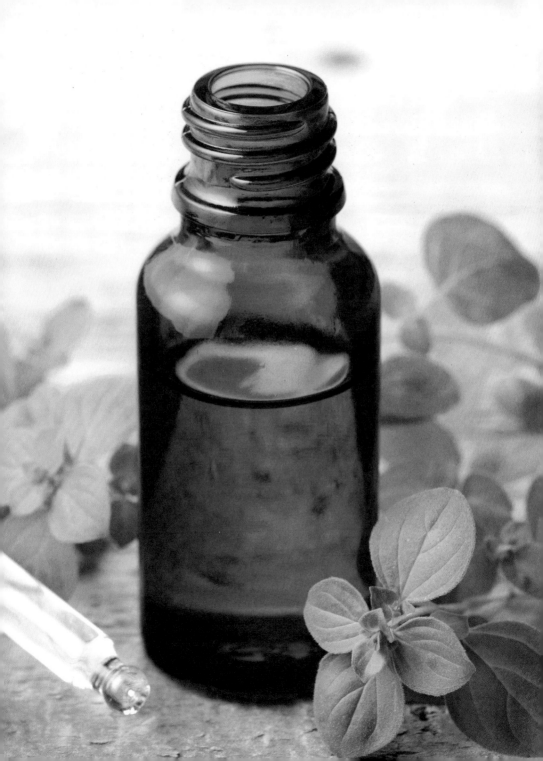

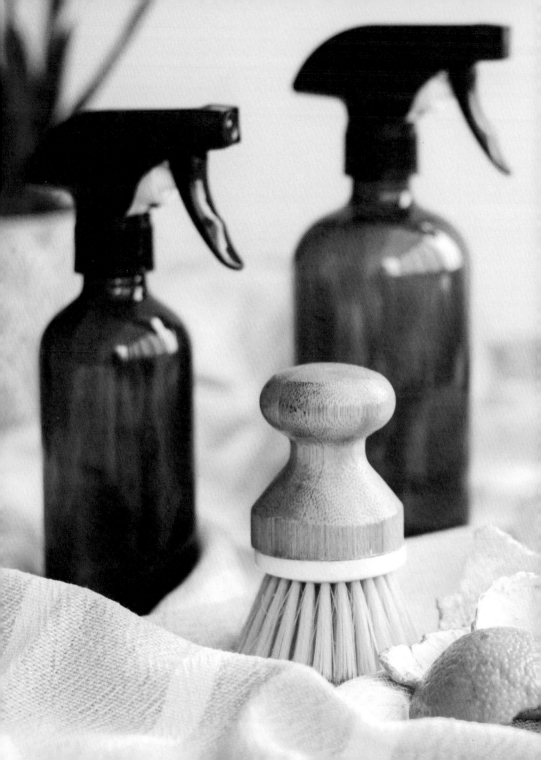

Orange Peel Vinegar Spritz

This spray cleaner smells amazing, and can be used almost anywhere in the house. Freshen up the kitchen table or countertops, sanitize cooking surfaces, clear up glass or mirrors, or degrease ceramic stove tops.

Ingredients:

1 cup Orange Peel Vinegar (see page 31)

1 cup distilled water

1   In a 16 OZ. spray bottle, add the ingredients and shake gently to combine.

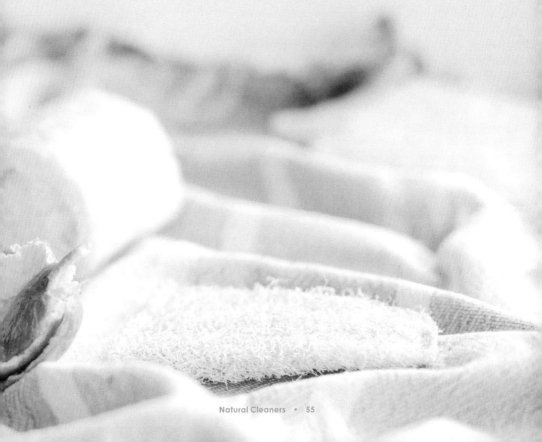

Washing Soda

The oven time will vary depending on how much you make, your oven's quirks, and what kind of pan(s) you're using; adjust for future batches accordingly. For more on washing soda, see page 18.

Ingredients:

2 lbs. baking soda

1 Preheat the oven to 400°F.

2 In a cake pan or oven pan, spread the baking soda in an even layer and place the pan in the oven.

3 Stirring occasionally, bake for at least 1 hour. What you're looking for is a flatter, grittier consistency, and a more yellowish color.

4 Allow it to cool, then store in a sealed container in a cool, dark place until ready to use.

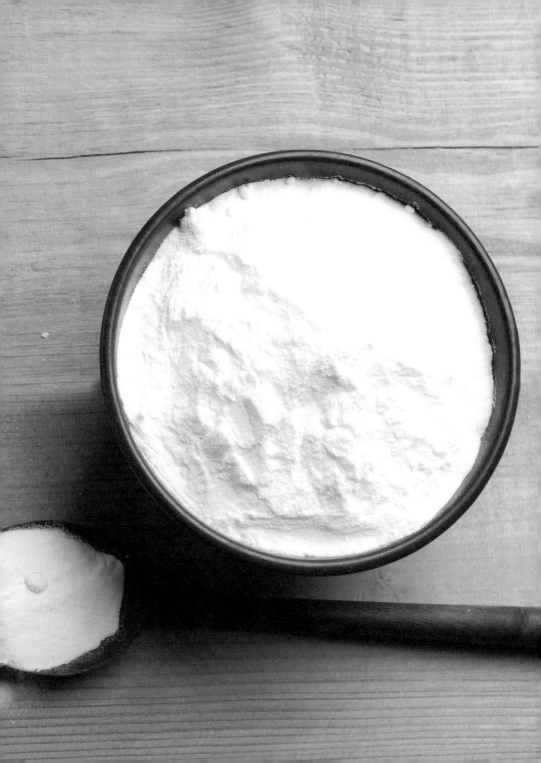

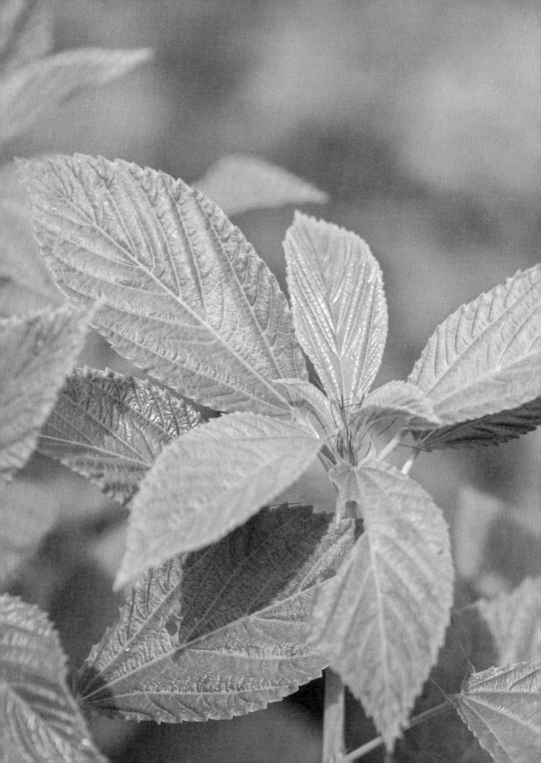

Oregano Scouring Powder

Use this powder on a predampened surface that can withstand scrubbing and scouring (i.e., not a glass cooktop). Use a brush to brighten up the grout in your tile work, or use it to clean your toilets. Feel free to experiment with different herbs—lavender and eucalyptus are obvious choices, but tea tree and lemon would serve well too.

Ingredients:

1½ cups baking soda

½ cup Washing Soda (see page 56)

2½ tablespoons liquid castile soap or True Liquid Castile Soap (see page 41)

1 tablespoon bruised fresh oregano

15 drops oregano essential oil

1   In a stainless steel or glass bowl, combine the baking soda and Washing Soda. While adding the dry ingredients, slowly fold in the liquid castile soap, stirring and fluffing with a fork to combine.

2   Add the herbs and essential oil and combine in the same way.

3   Store in a sealed jar until ready to use. To use, apply the powder to a damp surface, allow 5 minutes for it to work, then scrub.

Lemon-Eucalyptus Deep-Cleaning Scrubbing Paste

Tile floors, bathtubs, toilet bowls, stained pots and pans—when you need to go the extra mile to get something clean, this scrub is your friend. The essential oil blend used here makes for a very "clean" scent; experiment with other combos if you'd like!

Ingredients:

¾ cup baking soda

¼ cup liquid castile soap or True Liquid Castile Soap (see page 41)

5 drops lemon essential oil

5 drops eucalyptus essential oil

Distilled white vinegar, for cloth

1   In an 8 OZ. wide-mouth jar or plastic container, add the ingredients and stir with a spoon, knife, or chopstick to combine into a paste.

2   Using a brush, sponge, or cloth rag, apply the scrub to your chosen surface and work it in. Allow it to work for 10 or so minutes.

3   Wipe it away with a distilled white vinegar–dabbed rag or microfiber cloth.

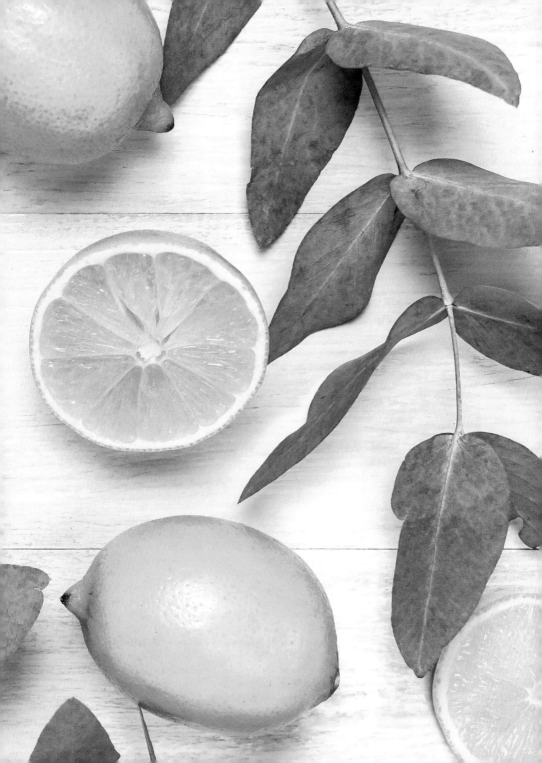

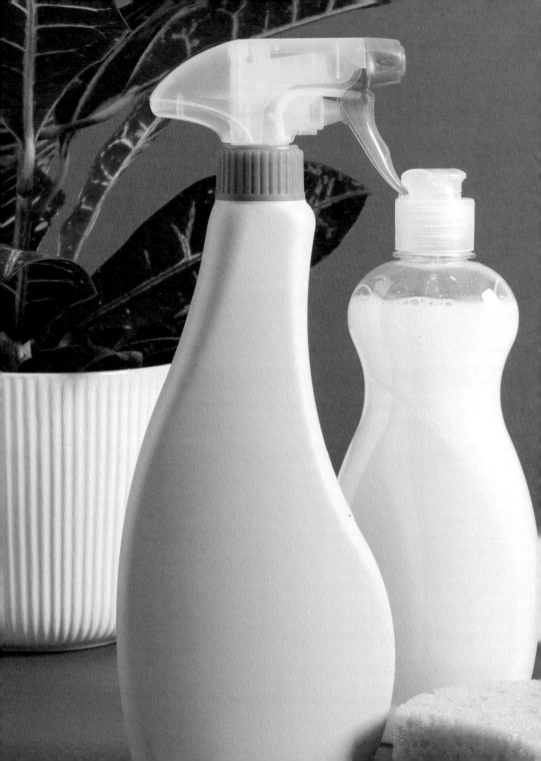

Grease & Grime Cleaner

If you have some nasty spills or grimy messes on hard surfaces—like in that area behind your trash can or behind the toilet—and you want to spray it away, this is a good option. Combining washing soda and castile soap makes for a hardworking spray.

Ingredients:

¼ cup Washing Soda (see page 56)

3½ cups distilled water

¼ cup liquid castile soap or True Liquid Castile Soap (see page 41)

1   Add the Washing Soda, then the distilled water, and then the soap to a 32 OZ. spray bottle and shake gently.

2   Spray the area you wish to clean and wait for a few minutes.

3   While wearing rubber kitchen gloves, wipe the area clean with microfiber cloths or cloth rags.

Cutting Board Cleaner

The salt grinds away accumulated gunk, while the acidic juice from the lemon disinfects. You'll finish with a spruced-up board ready for the next meal's ingredients.

Ingredients:

¼ cup salt

1 lemon, halved

1   Sprinkle the salt over your cutting board.

2   Use the lemon to scrub the cutting board vigorously. Allow the lemon-juice-and-salt mixture to remain on the board for a few minutes before rinsing and drying it.

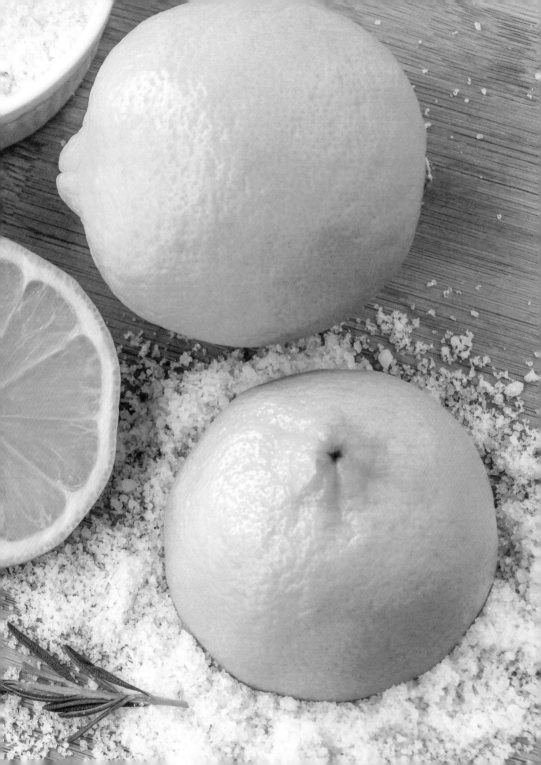

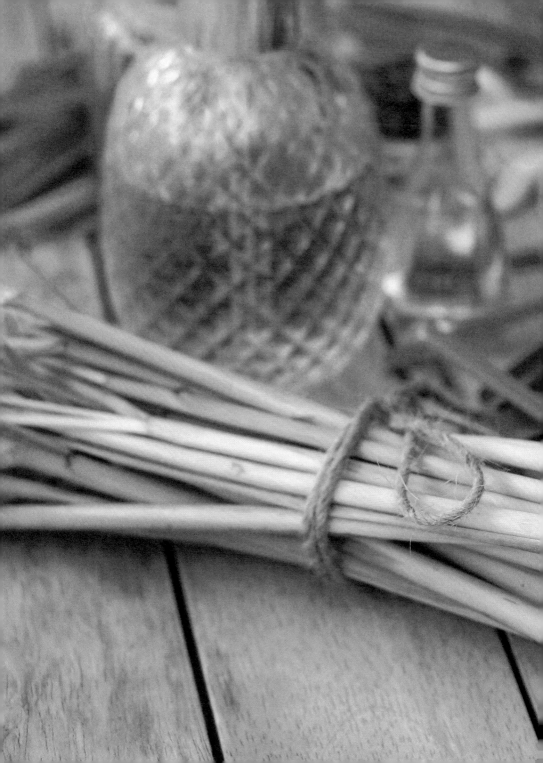

Cutting Board & Wooden Kitchen Utensil Conditioner

This wood conditioner can be customized with your choice of essential oil(s). Recondition your wooden kitchen utensils and cutting board every other month or whenever you want to add a shine to them. You can also use this to condition the butcher block.

Ingredients:

1½ cups virgin coconut oil

½ cup beeswax pellets

8 drops lemongrass essential oil

1   Set up your double boiler (see page 21) over low heat.

2   Add the coconut oil and beeswax and stir gently until they melt and combine, then immediately remove from heat.

3   Add the essential oil, stir, and pour into a 16 OZ. jar.

4   Seal the jar and store until ready for use. To use, apply the conditioner using a clean cloth.

Carefree Produce Spray

Not every market or grocery store has a full selection of affordable organic fruits and vegetables available, and you might have to buy produce that was treated with pesticides and wax. That's where this spray comes in, to remove those substances from the produce you intend to eat.

Ingredients:

2 cups distilled water

2 teaspoons liquid castile soap or True Liquid Castile Soap (see page 41)

1 In a 16 OZ. spray bottle, add the distilled water and then the castile soap. Shake gently to combine. Be sure to shake before every use.

2 Spray your produce thoroughly before serving it, massaging the solution into the skin or leaves. For root vegetables, consider using a scrub brush as well.

3 Wait 10 to 20 seconds, then rinse thoroughly.

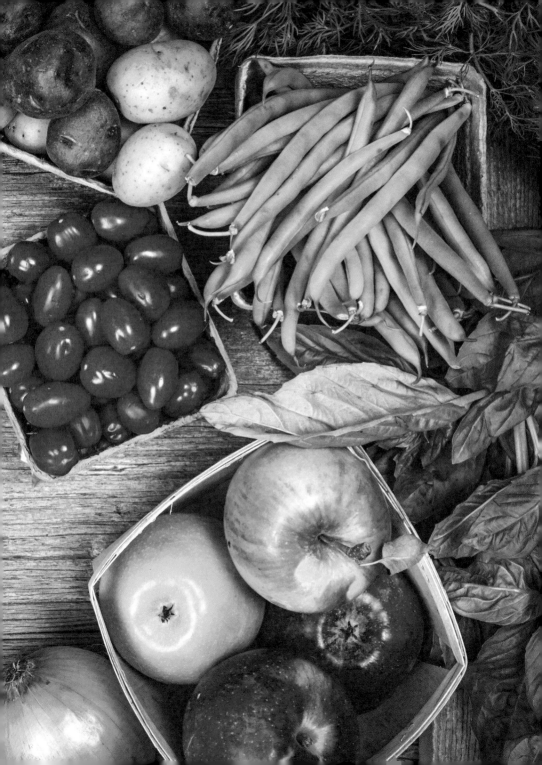

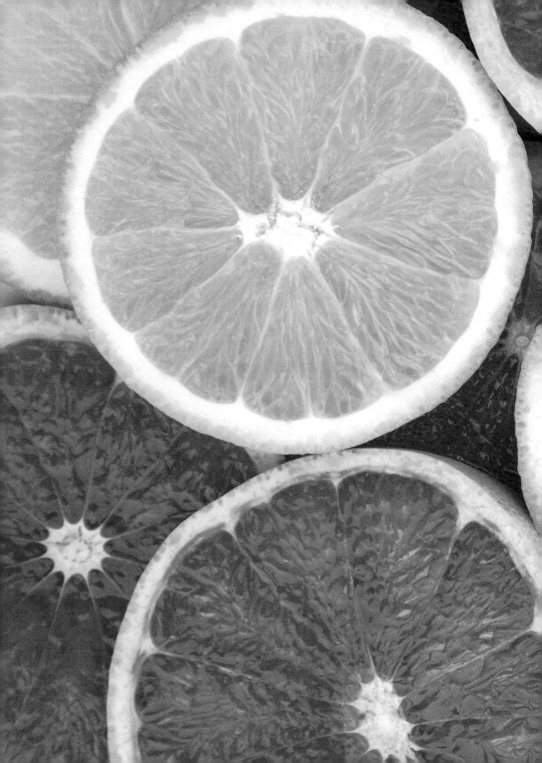

Citrus Punch Hand-Wash & Dish Soap

If you're just cleaning up after a single meal, or if you don't have a dishwasher, this all-natural and easy dish soap recipe will get the job done. Infused with grapefruit and orange essential oils, it will also liven up your chore time! Note: don't use this soap in a dishwasher.

Ingredients:

5 cups distilled water

½ cup liquid castile soap or True Liquid Castile Soap (see page 41)

5 drops grapefruit essential oil

5 drops orange essential oil

1. Add the distilled water to your dish soap dispenser, then add the remaining ingredients.

2. Shake moderately, until fully combined, and use. Give the soap a gentle shake before each use.

Dishwasher Powder Detergent

You might find citric acid powder in your local supermarket's baking or canning aisle, or at a big-box store in your area. If you don't have any luck there, you can order non-GMO citric acid powder online, and it can be on your doorstep in a few days. Consider getting extra so you can make a bigger batch of detergent, if you'd like.

Ingredients:

1 cup Washing Soda (see page 56)

¼ cup salt

½ cup citric acid powder

20 drops lemon essential oil

1   In a mixing bowl, combine all of the ingredients with a fork.

2   Store in an airtight 16 OZ. glass jar and seal. Store in a cool, dark, dry place until ready to use.

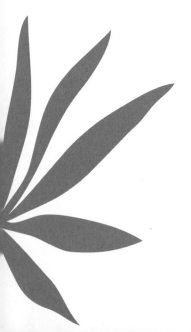

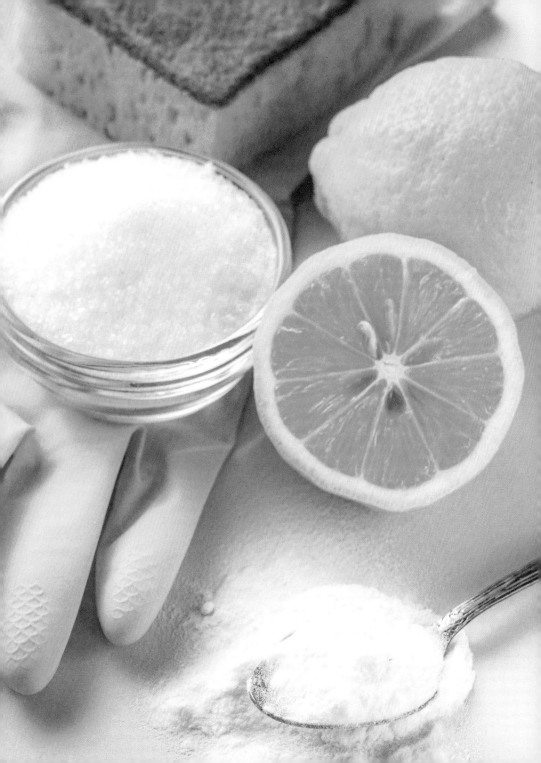

Natural Dishwasher Rinse Aid

Instead of using commercial rinse aids in your dishwasher, which are chock-full of chemicals, try this recipe. Unlike a vinegar-based formula, it won't eat away at the rubber dishwasher parts over time.

Ingredients:

¼ cup 3% hydrogen peroxide

6 drops lemon essential oil

1   Run your dishwasher several times without adding a commercial rinse aid, to clear out any chemicals from the dispenser.

2   Add the hydrogen peroxide, then the essential oil, to the dispenser and run the dishwasher.

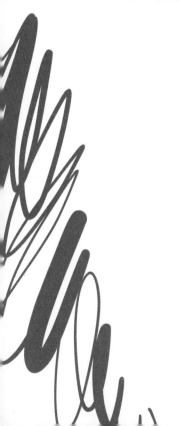

Glass Stove Top Cleaner

When the pot marks and water stains can't be ignored any longer, go over your entire glass stove top with this cleaner to restore the shine. If you want to prevent this scenario from happening in the first place, or at least try to, use the screen cleaner on page 87 for a quick daily wipe-down.

Ingredients:

1 cup warm water

1 cup baking soda

1 Add the water to a 8 OZ. spray bottle and spritz the entire stove top surface.

2 Sprinkle the baking soda on evenly, aiming to cover the whole stove top.

3 Spray the warm water again to wet the baking soda. If your spray bottle runs out of water before all of the baking soda is wet, refill your bottle and continue spraying. Let it sit for 15 minutes.

4 Use a clean rag or microfiber cloth to scrub the stove top, then wipe the baking soda away. Repeat the process as needed.

5 Wipe dry with a fresh cloth towel, rag, or microfiber cloth.

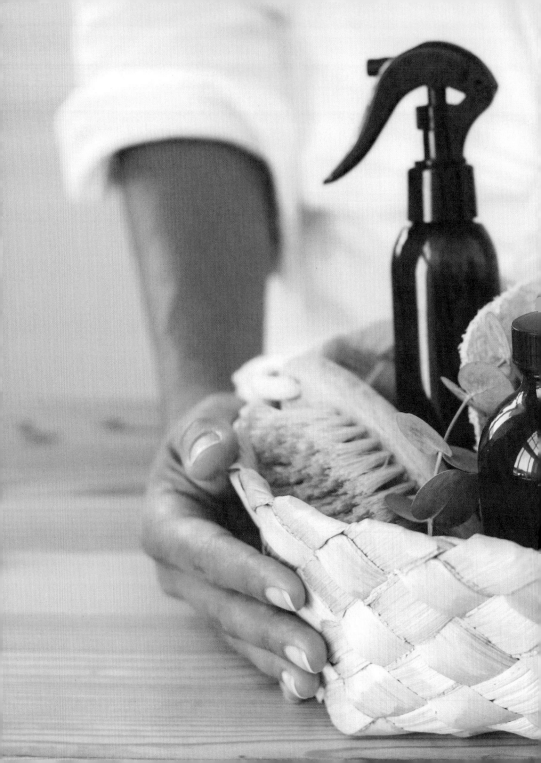

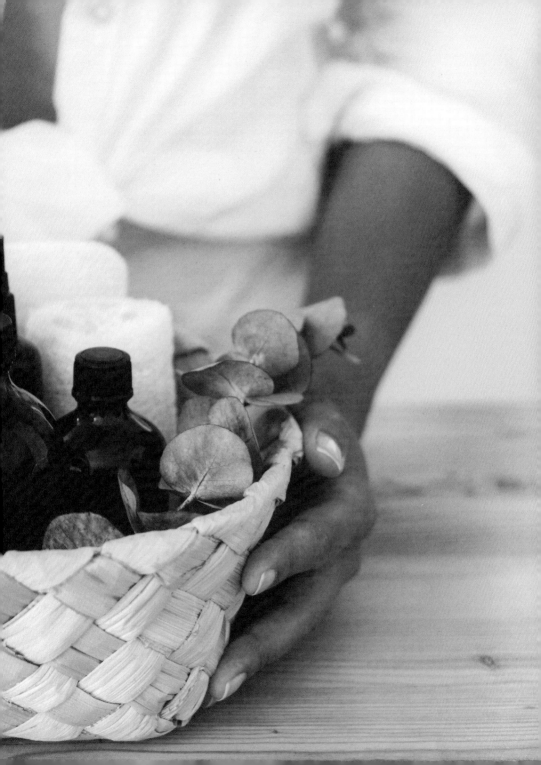

Oven Cleaner

Commercial oven cleaners contain some of the harshest chemicals you can find in a grocery store. In fact, of the 13 oven cleaner products ranked by the Environmental Working Group, 12 got Fs! Switching to this extremely simple recipe is a quick and easy step toward detoxing your home.

Ingredients:

6 tablespoons baking soda

3 tablespoons distilled water

1 to 2 splashes distilled white vinegar, for cloth

1   In a bowl, add the baking soda. Add the distilled water and stir to make a paste.

2   Using a cloth rag, sponge, brush, or even your hands, spread the paste onto the surfaces inside the oven. This includes the glass window, but does not include any reachable heating coils or burners.

3   Give the paste at least half an hour and up to a whole day to work. Then wipe clean with rags or microfiber cloths dabbed with the vinegar.

Grill Grate & Oven Rack Cleaning Treatment

Depending on what foods you're cooking and how often you're cleaning your grill, grill grates can get pretty dirty. The same goes for oven racks, probably to a lesser extent. This recipe is for that once-in-a-while reset. You'll need a big container—a plastic storage tote will do.

Ingredients:

Several gallons hot water

3 cups Washing Soda (see page 56)

1   Add enough hot water to completely submerge your grill racks or grates in a large tub or tote.

2   Pour in the Washing Soda and stir to mix.

3   Allow it to sit all day or overnight.

4   Scrub the grate or racks with a mesh pad or brush.

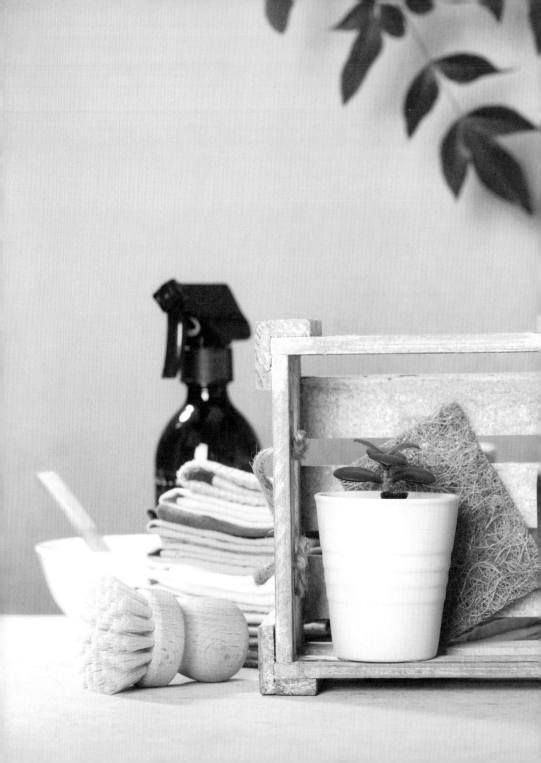

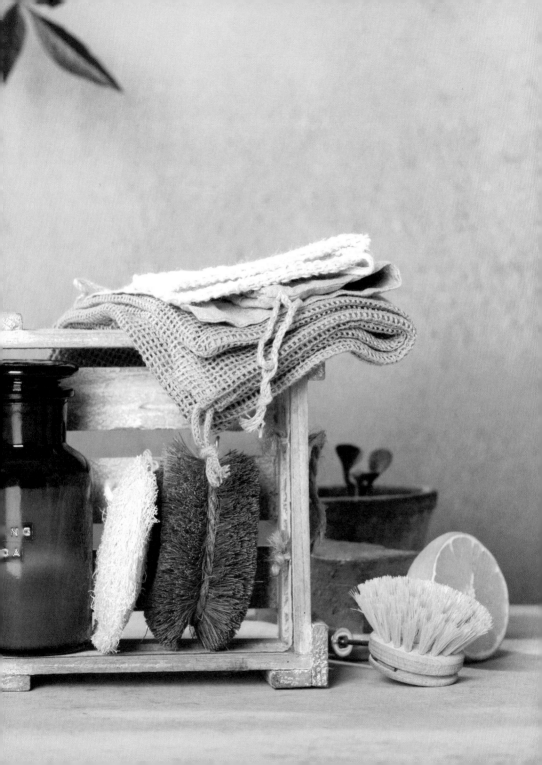

Stainless Steel Appliance Cleaner

If your stainless steel appliances are fingerprint resistant, then you should never use even mildly harsh cleaners—including baking soda and vinegar—or rub or wipe them with sponges or harsh cloths. This gentle recipe will work without damaging the fingerprint-resistant coating.

Ingredients:

2 tablespoons liquid castile soap or True Liquid Castile Soap (see page 41)

4 cups warm water

1 In a kitchen bucket or large bowl, pour the soap, then add the warm water.

2 Wet a clean, soft cotton towel, rag, or microfiber cloth in the bucket and gently wipe down the appliance(s) in a circular motion.

3 To avoid streaks, dry with a fresh cloth or towel.

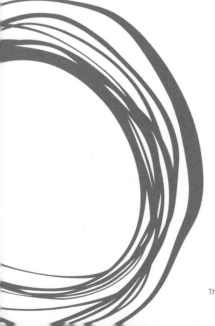

Clog Remover & Drain Cleaner

There are many ways to clear clogged drains without resorting to commercial chemical drain cleaners—which is for the best, because those products are some of the nastiest you can find on supermarket shelves. Be sure to prevent clogs in the first place by placing catchers over the drains in your showers, tubs, and sinks, and keep a plunger and drum auger/drain snake handy to mechanically clear drains.

Ingredients:

1 cup Washing Soda (see page 56)

3 cups boiling water

1 Pour the Washing Soda into your clogged drain.

2 Pour the boiling water into the drain and leave it for at least half an hour.

3 Rinse and repeat as needed.

THE BAKING SODA & VINEGAR METHOD

Here's an alternative drain cleaner. Try both and see which one you prefer.

Ingredients:

1 cup baking soda

1 cup hot water

1 cup vinegar

1 Pour the baking soda into your clogged drain.

2 Mix the water and vinegar, then pour the mixture into the drain.

3 Plug the drain and fill the sink or tub with hot water and wait 5 minutes.

4 Unplug the drain to flush out the pipe. Repeat as necessary.

Lemon Juice Descaler

Limescale, aka calcium carbonate ($CaCO_3$), is a hard, white, metallic substance that mucks up sinks, showerheads, dishwashers, toilets, washing machines, coffee carafes—anywhere that hard water containing dissolved calcium and magnesium molecules flows hot and evaporates. Luckily there's an easy, natural way to get rid of it: lemon juice.

Washing Machine

Add 1 cup of lemon juice instead of laundry detergent and run the machine once when there are no clothes in it.

Dishwasher

Splash 1 cup of lemon juice in the bottom of the dishwasher and run the machine when there are no dishes in it.

Drip Coffee Maker

Add ½ cup of lemon juice to your coffee maker's water reservoir, and fill it the rest of the way with water. Run the coffee maker without coffee or a filter. Throw out the lemon water, then rinse by running the coffee maker with just water until it's ready to go again.

Faucets & Fixtures

Soak clean rags or cloths in lemon juice and, using rubber bands, wrap the cloth around the affected metal. The trick is to keep the lemon juice on the limescale for at least an hour. After an hour or two, remove the cloths and scrub away the limescale.

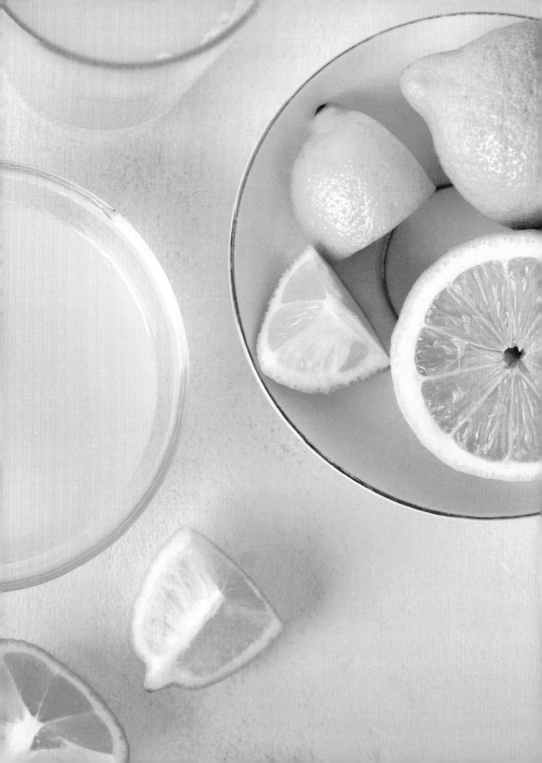

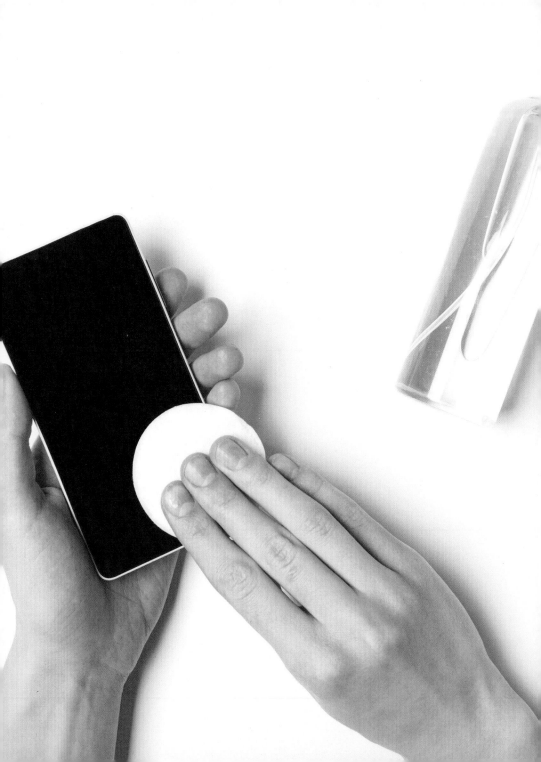

Screen Cleaner

If you can make it a habit to clean all of the screens—laptops, desktops, tablets, phones, TVs—in your home and office (or home office) in one go, you'll save so much time. This recipe uses vinegar instead of alcohol, because alcohol can eat away at screen materials; distilled water won't leave a residue on your screen like tap water will. If you want to make a different quantity, the formula is 1:1 vinegar to water.

Ingredients:

1 cup distilled water

1 cup distilled white vinegar

1 In a 16 OZ. spray bottle, combine the ingredients and shake gently.

2 Spray the cleaner onto a microfiber cloth or reusable cotton round. For larger screens, spray the screen itself if preferred.

3 Wipe the microfiber cloth gently across the screen and let it air dry.

Window Cleaner

Cleaning the windows in your home or car is simple (and easier on the lungs than conventional window cleaner) when you use this recipe. If you want a different scent, just substitute a neutral dish soap (or drop dish soap from the recipe entirely) and add 5 to 10 drops of your preferred essential oil(s).

Ingredients:

1 cup distilled water

1 cup distilled white vinegar

1 dash Citrus Punch Hand-Wash & Dish Soap (see page 71)

1   In a 16 OZ. spray bottle, add the ingredients and shake gently to combine.

2   On a cloudy day or when the sun's not bright on your glass, spray your windows liberally and wait 1 to 2 minutes.

3   Working from the top down, use a microfiber cloth to wipe the windows clean.

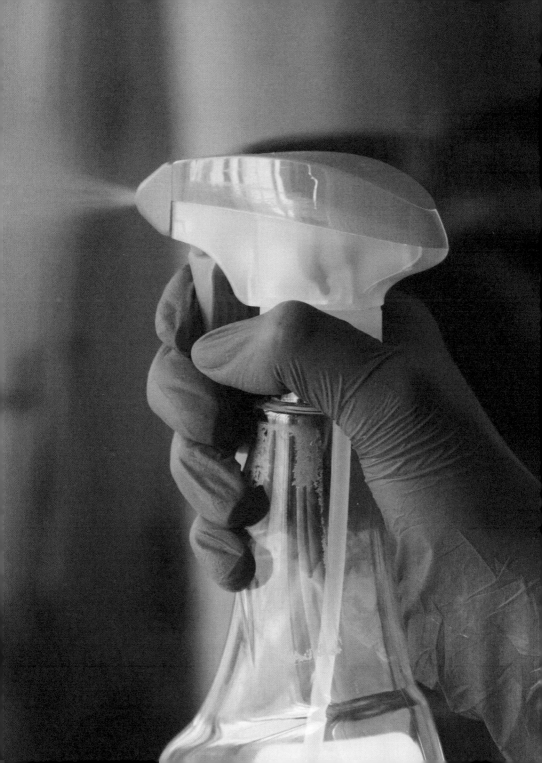

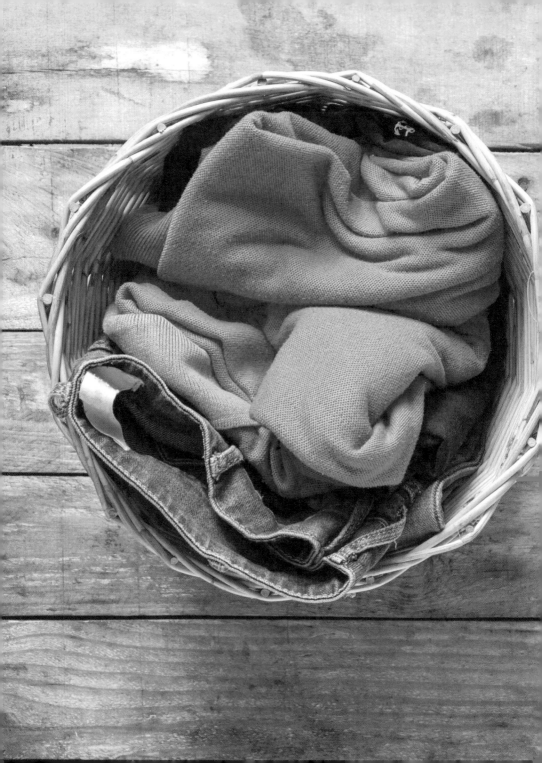

Laundry Stain Remover

You probably have an idea of which items of clothing you'll need to pretreat before your next wash (at least the clothes you personally wore). Those items—the ketchup-stained T-shirt from the barbecue, the coffee-stained pants from when you hit a bump while taking a sip in the car—are what this recipe is for.

Ingredients:

½ cup Washing Soda (see page 56)

¾ cup warm water

¼ cup vinegar

1   Sprinkle the Washing Soda on the stain.

2   In an 8 to 16 OZ. spray bottle, mix the water and vinegar.

3   Spray the Washing Soda area and let it sit for 15 minutes. Fold a different part of the garment or linen over to scrub the area, or use a soft toothbrush, if desired. Then toss the item into the wash with the rest of the laundry.

Rosemary Liquid Laundry Detergent

If cedarwood, lavender, or lemon scents sound more appealing (and those are all great choices for a clean laundry smell), simply substitute as preferred.

Ingredients:

2 cups baking soda

⅔ cup fine sea salt

4 cups hot water

2 cups liquid castile soap or True Liquid Castile Soap (see page 41)

20 drops rosemary essential oil

1   In a 1-gallon glass jug, add the dry ingredients, and then the water. Close the jug and shake until the baking soda and salt are dissolved.

2   Add the castile soap and essential oil and shake until fully mixed.

3   Shake before use and pour ¼ cup into the machine for a regular load.

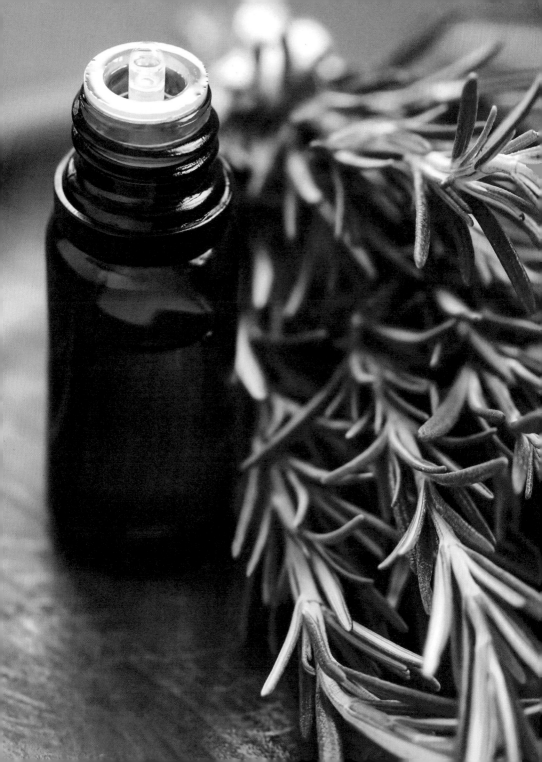

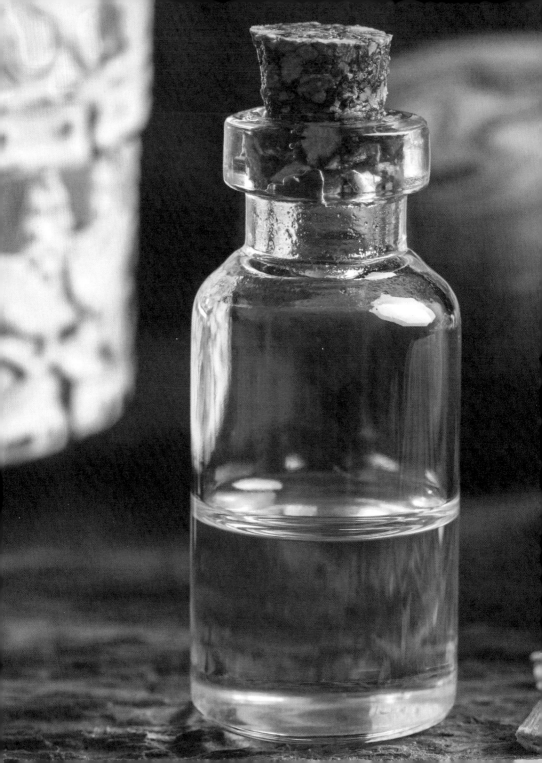

Cedarwood-Clove
Laundry Detergent Powder

This recipe will make your clothes smell spicy and woodsy. Feel free to play around with other essential oil blends too. When you're ready to do laundry, toss 1 tablespoon directly on the clothes for light loads, and up to 3 tablespoons for heavy or especially dirty loads.

Ingredients:

1 (4 OZ.) bar unscented castile soap

1 lb. baking soda

3½ lbs. Washing Soda (see page 56)

15 drops cedarwood essential oil

10 drops clove essential oil

1   Use a cheese grater to finely grate the bar of castile soap. The more surface area, the better.

2   In a bucket or large bowl, mix the dry ingredients together and stir in the essential oils.

3   Store in a large, sealable container or in multiple smaller containers in a dry place until ready to use.

Eucalyptus–Tea Tree Carpet Spray

After enlisting your family's help in picking up, go to town with this easy-to-make spray cleaner, and the result will be an incredibly clean-smelling carpet. Repeat every other week or as needed.

Ingredients:

1½ cups vinegar

2 cups distilled water

2 teaspoons fine salt

5 drops eucalyptus essential oil

15 drops tea tree essential oil

1 Add the vinegar and distilled water to a 32 OZ. spray bottle and shake to combine.

2 Add the salt and essential oils and shake to combine.

3 Spray the entire carpet or rug, shaking the spray bottle often, hitting particularly dirty areas hardest.

4 Allow it to rest for 15 minutes, then vacuum the carpet or rug as normal.

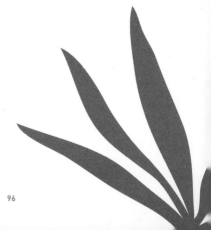

Carpet Stain Remover

When a routine area spritz and vacuuming won't finish off a tough stain, it's time to power up. The combo of baking soda and vinegar brings the chemistry magic.

Ingredients:

¼ cup baking soda

¼ cup distilled water

10 drops grapefruit essential oil

¼ cup distilled white vinegar

1   In a small bowl, mix the baking soda into the distilled water and then pour or funnel the mixture into an 8 OZ. spray bottle.

2   Add the essential oil and vinegar, cap, and shake.

3   Spray the stain liberally and let the cleaner work for up to half an hour.

4   Spritz the stain lightly again and, using a clean scrub brush or cloth, depending on how deep the stain is, scrub and work the stain out. Vacuum afterward or allow it to air dry.

Lavender-Lemon Carpet & Rug Deodorizer Powder

Baking soda absorbs odors, while lavender fights microbes and lemon brightens a room's energy. This recipe can work in tandem with the Eucalyptus–Tea Tree Carpet Spray (see page 96).

Ingredients:

2 cups baking soda

25 drops lavender essential oil

10 drops lemon essential oil

1   In a 16 OZ. sealable jar or a parmesan cheese shaker, add the ingredients and shake to combine.

2   If using a jar, create a lid with holes—wax paper with holes punched using a pen is one option.

3   Shake the powder over the entire rug or carpet and let it sit overnight, or throughout the day while everyone is at work or school.

4   Vacuum until the powder is completely sucked up.

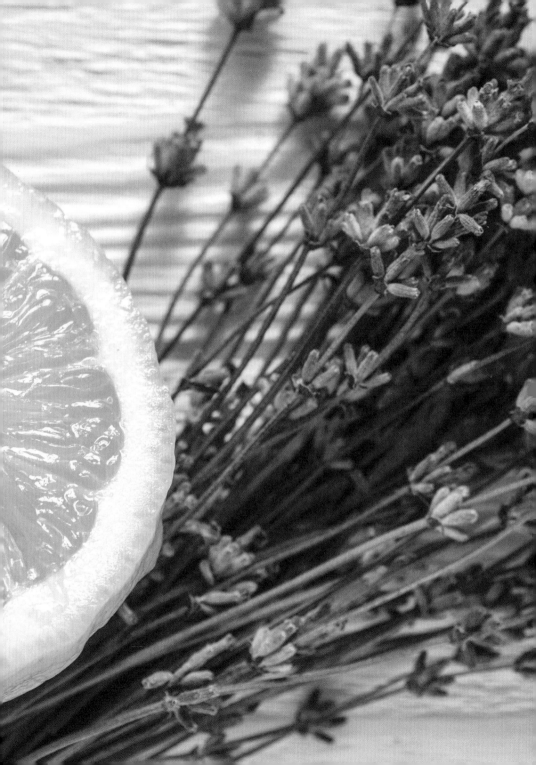

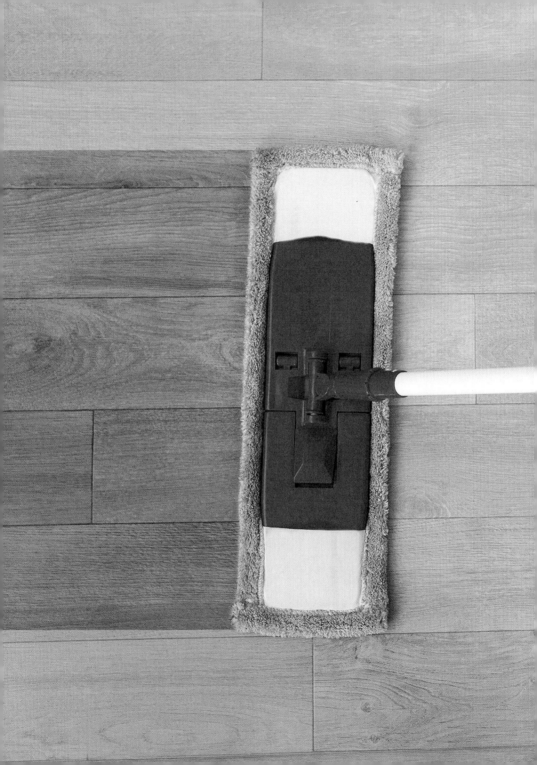

Hardwood Floor Restorer

If you have nice hardwood floors, then no doubt they are a focal point for your home, and you want to keep them beautiful and well maintained. This recipe gives an old-world shine to any hardwood floor. And since it's made from natural ingredients, the used mop water can be safely discarded on weeds you'd like to knock back, or just down the drain.

Ingredients:

1 cup vinegar

1 cup extra-virgin olive oil

Juice of 2 lemons

8 cups warm water

1   In a clean bucket, combine the ingredients.

2   Use a cloth mop to apply the solution to the hardwood floor, gently mopping.

3   Open your windows and/or set up fans to blow the floor dry. Alternatively, wring your mop into a dry bucket and soak up the floor restorer with the mop.

Air Freshener

If you're using a different size jar or container, adjust your ingredients accordingly. Make one for the car as well and set the container in one of the cup holders.

Ingredients:

6 tablespoons baking soda

10 drops lemon essential oil

10 drops eucalyptus essential oil

1 Add the baking soda and then the essential oils to a bowl or a 4 OZ. wide-mouth jar and seal the container.

2 Shake, then remove the lid.

3 Cover the container's opening with a piece of tea towel or other linen, cotton, or muslin cloth. Secure the cloth with a jar lid ring or a rubber band.

4 To use, set in a location of your preference.

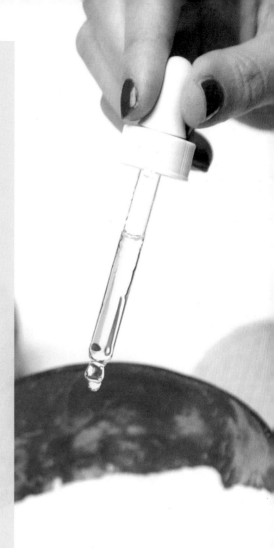

EASY CAR FRESHENERS FOR AC VENTS

Try this in addition to or instead of the Air Freshener recipe for your car or office or at home if you have a window or portable air conditioner. Play with the essential oil blends to find your preferred scent.

Ingredients:

2 wooden clothespins

20 drops clove essential oil

20 drops sweet orange essential oil

1   In a dish or plastic container, set the clothespins on their sides.

2   Add the essential oils and allow the oils to soak into the wood for a few hours.

3   Flip the clothespins over and allow it to set overnight.

4   Allow the clothespins to dry out, then clip them to vents in your car or on your portable AC unit.

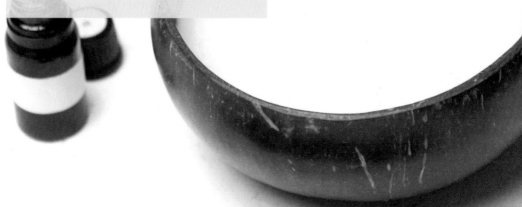

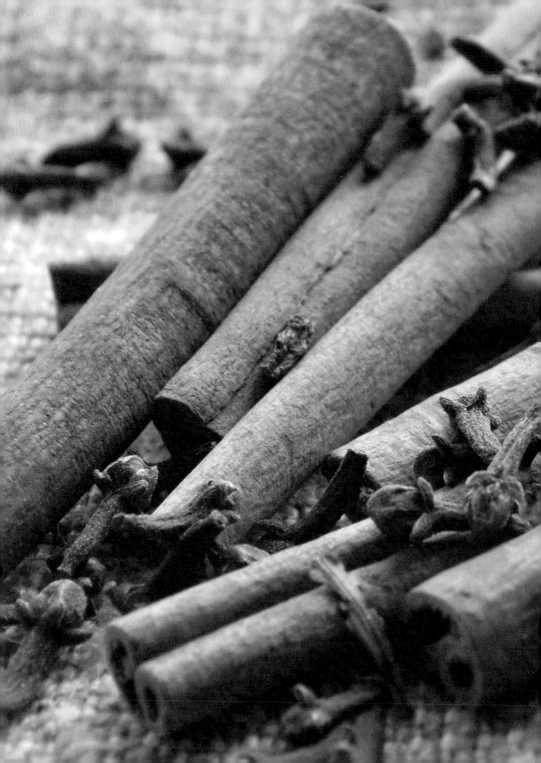

Guest Room Linen Mist

If you have friends or family coming for a visit, a very easy way to make them feel right at home is to show them to a room with clean linens and a fresh aroma—in this case, of clove and cinnamon—in the air. Play with the essential oil blends as you like.

Ingredients:

½ cup distilled water

30 drops cinnamon essential oil (cassia, bark, and leaf all work)

15 drops clove essential oil

1 In a 4 OZ. mister bottle, add the distilled water and then the essential oils and shake gently to mix.

2 An hour or two before your guests arrive, mist the linens, flooring, curtains, and center of the room to your liking.

Tile & Grout Cleaner

This recipe couldn't be more basic: just mix washing soda and warm water. You'll want rubber gloves and your favorite scrubbing brush to get the job done. But the end result—a sparkling, naturally clean bathroom or kitchen—will be well worth the effort. This will also work on your porcelain and ceramic fixtures: toilet, sink, tub, etc.

Ingredients:	½ cup Washing Soda (see page 56)
	1 gallon warm water

1 In a 1-gallon bucket, add the Washing Soda, then the warm water, and stir with a wooden spoon to combine.

2 Apply to the whole area you wish to clean and begin scrubbing immediately.

3 Wipe up with warm, wet towels.

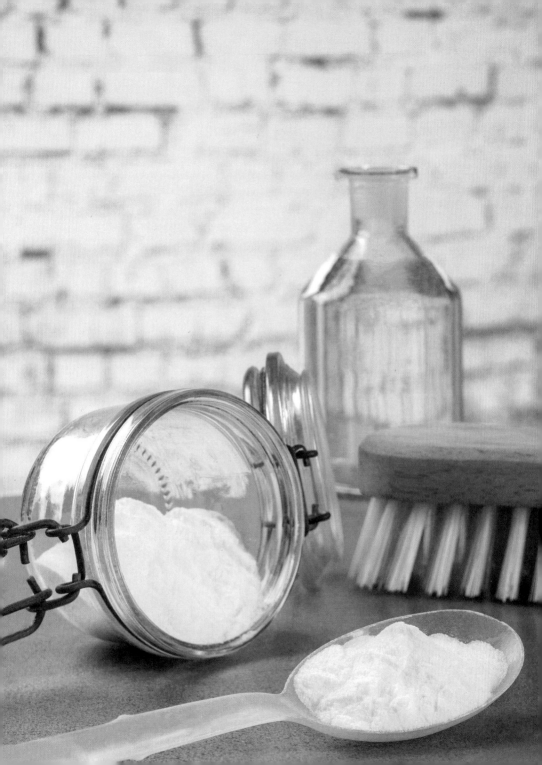

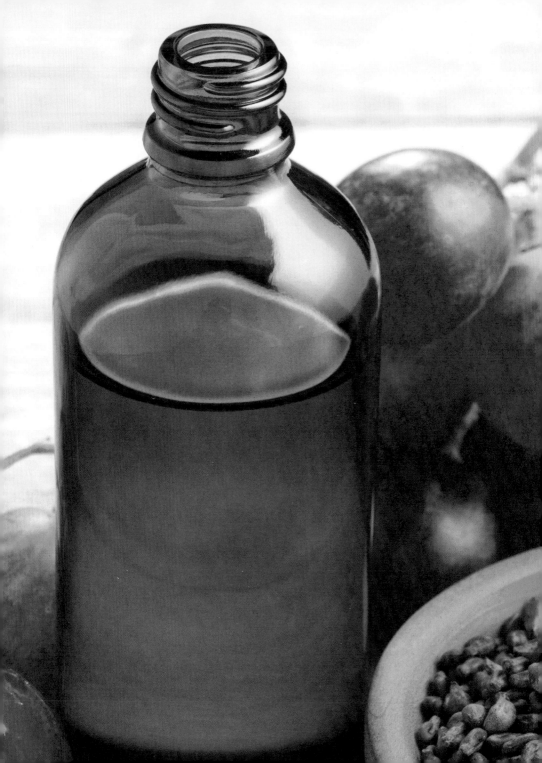

Car Upholstery Cleaner & Protectant

If you're like most people, you spend a lot of time in your car. Why not make sure your car's air quality is good for you too? Try this recipe instead of the prevailing commercial protectant, so you don't get stuck breathing in harsh chemicals.

Ingredients:

1 cup distilled water

1 cup organic grapeseed oil

1 tablespoon Orange Peel Vinegar (see page 31)

1   In a 16 OZ. spray bottle, add all of the ingredients and shake gently to combine.

2   Either spray directly on your car's leather or vinyl upholstery, console, dashboard, and so on, or spray generously onto a clean cloth, rag, or microfiber cloth.

3   Wipe in circular motions until the upholstery shines.

Garage & Outdoor Hardscaping Wash

If you have a wet stain on a concrete surface, use clay-based cat litter or sawdust to soak it up overnight and then discard. But if it's a dry or stubborn stain, keep reading! This recipe also helps to deep clean patio pavers, driveways, and other hardscaped walkways. For serious stains, sprinkle a cup of washing soda over the stained area and let it sit overnight before proceeding.

Ingredients:

2 cups Washing Soda (see page 56)

4 gallons water

1 In a bucket set up outside or in a well-ventilated area, add the Washing Soda, then the water.

2 Pour or mop the mixture over the surface and allow it to sit for half an hour.

3 Using an outdoor push brush or large scrub brush, brush the area gently.

4 Rinse with water and allow it to air dry.

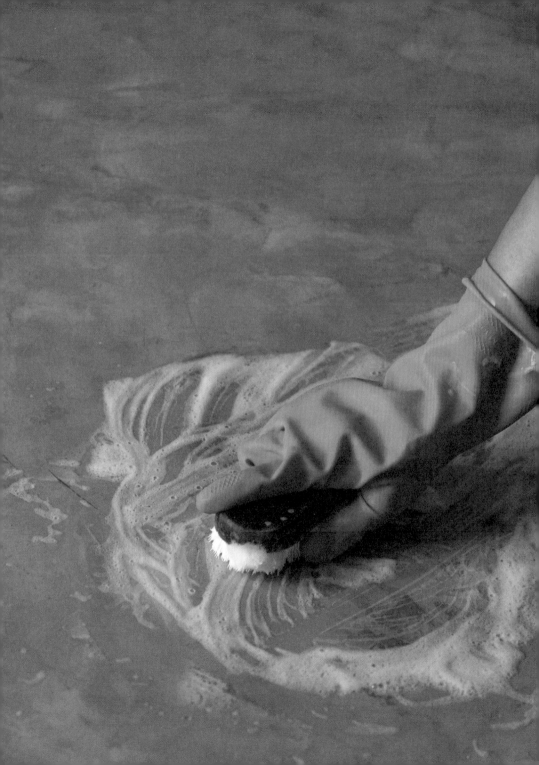

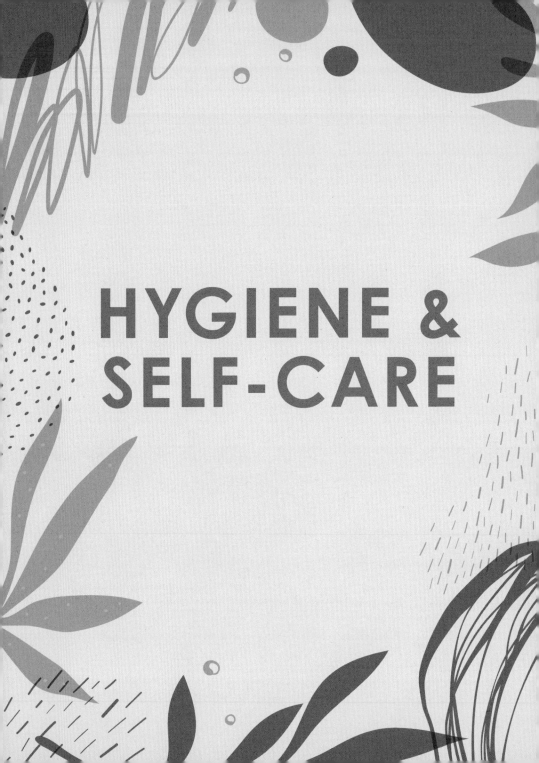

HYGIENE & SELF-CARE

With low-cost and long-lasting ingredients, these handmade care products will make you feel (and smell) great. Ditch the drugstore products and expensive treatments and embrace the natural healing properties of essential oils, apple cider vinegar, teas, shea butter, clays, oats, and more.

The following recipes introduce you to a full array of skin-care staples, body scrubs, lip balms, conditioners, and other DIY beauty products that will have you glowing.

Hoppy Deodorant

A deodorant you can trust to be chemical and aluminum free, plus one whose scent you can customize? What's not to love? You can buy BPA-free plastic deodorant stick containers online, or you can use jars or tins. The hops extract adds an extra antibacterial oomph.

Ingredients:

3 tablespoons coconut oil

2 tablespoons shea butter

3 tablespoons baking soda

2 tablespoons arrowroot powder

10 to 15 drops hops extract

Essential oils (see sidebar)

1   Set up a double boiler (see page 21) over low heat and add the coconut oil and shea butter.

2   As soon as the coconut oil and shea butter are fully melted, remove from heat and stir to mix.

3   Add the remaining ingredients and stir to combine.

4   Before the mixture cools, pour or spoon into your container(s) of choice and allow it to solidify completely. Store in a cool, dark place where the coconut oil won't melt (i.e., somewhere below 76°F) between uses.

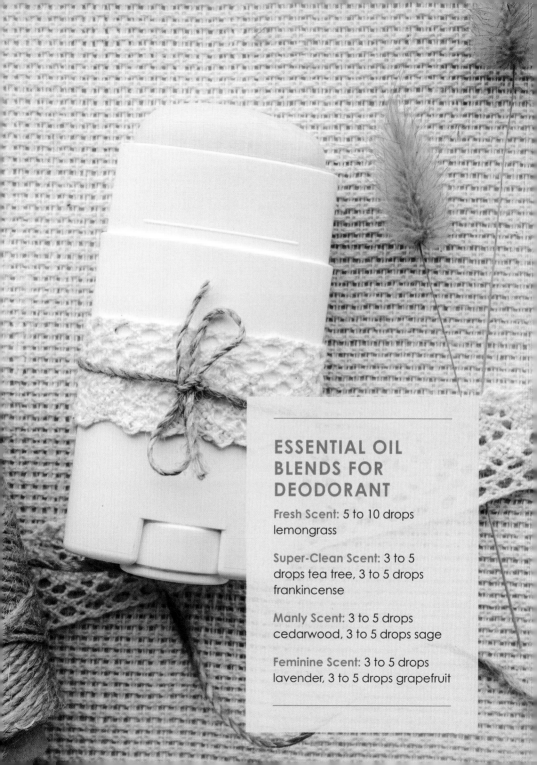

ESSENTIAL OIL BLENDS FOR DEODORANT

Fresh Scent: 5 to 10 drops lemongrass

Super-Clean Scent: 3 to 5 drops tea tree, 3 to 5 drops frankincense

Manly Scent: 3 to 5 drops cedarwood, 3 to 5 drops sage

Feminine Scent: 3 to 5 drops lavender, 3 to 5 drops grapefruit

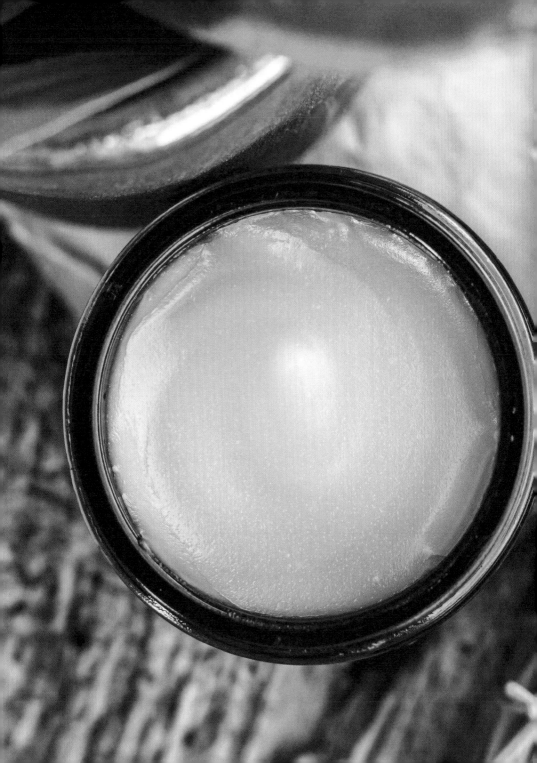

Ginger-Coconut Lip Balm

If you want to get really fancy, you can source your own lip balm tubes. For this recipe, a 4 OZ. jar or four 1 OZ. tins will do the trick. If you don't have sweet almond oil, just replace it with the same amount of coconut oil or jojoba oil. You can customize the essential oil to your liking.

Ingredients:

¼ cup coconut oil

2 tablespoons sweet almond oil

2 tablespoons beeswax

2 drops ginger essential oil, or your preferred oil

1   Set up your double boiler (see page 21) over low heat.

2   Add the coconut oil, sweet almond oil, and beeswax to the double boiler in order and stir slowly to melt the coconut oil and beeswax. Add the ginger essential oil.

3   Stir to combine and quickly remove from heat. Pour the wax mixture into your jar(s) and let it cool before using.

Clove-Peppermint Toothpaste

This toothpaste is easy to make and will make your mouth feel amazing. Clove oil strengthens teeth while lending a powerful, pleasant aromatic experience.

Ingredients:

4 tablespoons coconut oil

4 tablespoons baking soda

10 drops clove essential oil

10 drops peppermint essential oil

1   In a bowl or 4 OZ. glass jar, melt the coconut oil in 15-second increments in the microwave. Do not overcook it.

2   Mix in the baking soda thoroughly.

3   Add the essential oils and stir to combine, then allow the toothpaste to cool solid before using.

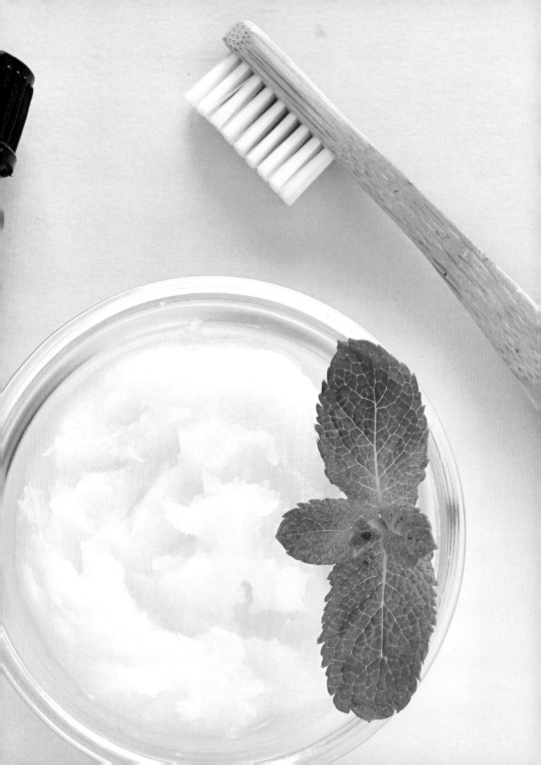

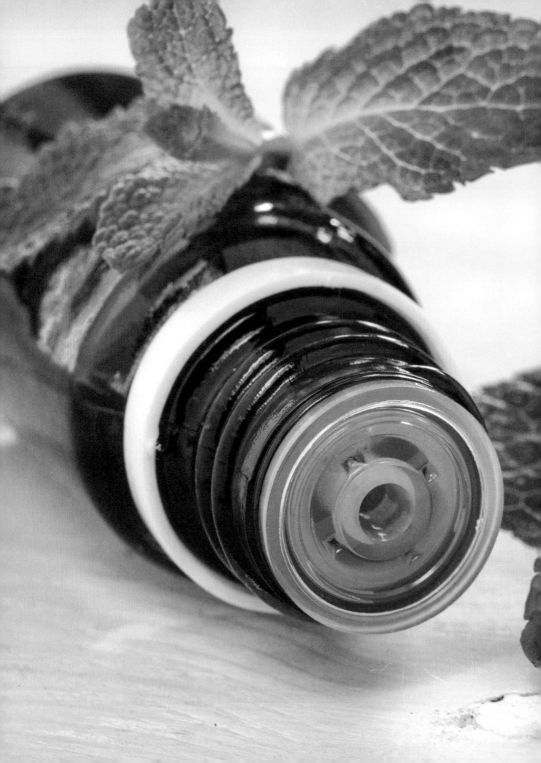

Tea Tree & Peppermint Mouthwash

Add this mouthwash to your nightly dental hygiene routine to take full advantage of tea tree oil's ability to fight germs, reduce inflammation, and rebuild gums. The peppermint adds a fresh feeling to your mouth.

Ingredients:

2 cups distilled water

2½ tablespoons baking soda

8 drops tea tree essential oil

8 drops peppermint essential oil

1 Combine all of the ingredients together in a glass jar and shake well.

2 To use, swish a mouthful for 30 seconds, gargling if desired, before spitting out.

Flaxseed Gel for Hair

Flaxseed gel nourishes hair and freshens up the scalp. It's especially good for those who have wavy or curly hair, because it adds body and structure. Use it as a hair mask, leaving it in your hair for 15 minutes before rinsing it out, or save for use in the Rosemary–Flaxseed Gel Shampoo (see page 125). You can also add herbs or essential oils to the gel itself.

Ingredients:

2 cups distilled water

¼ cup organic flaxseeds

1   In a pot on high heat, pour the distilled water and the flaxseeds and let the water come to a boil. Turn the heat to medium and stir continually.

2   Cook for about 5 more minutes, or until you see a slimy froth on the water.

3   Strain through a cheesecloth into a small jar. Using gloves or tongs, squeeze the cloth bag of flaxseeds to extract more gel into the jar.

4   Seal the jar and store it in the fridge, making sure to use the gel within two weeks.

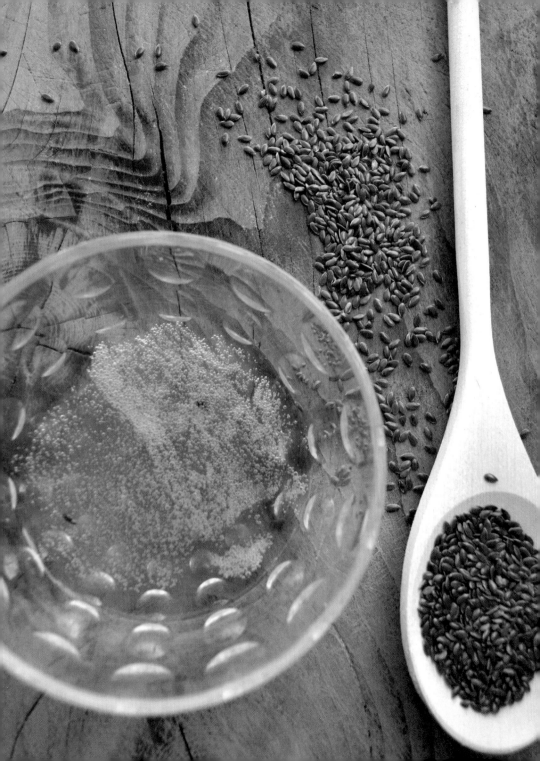

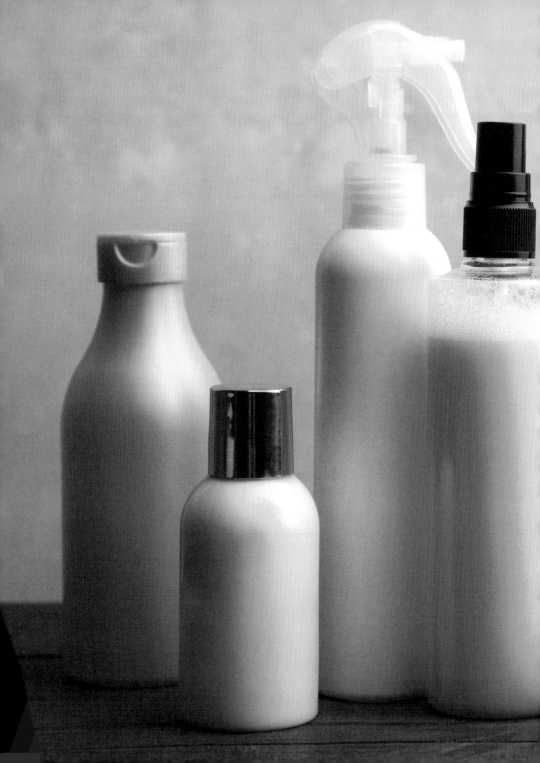

Rosemary–Flaxseed Gel Shampoo

Rich with antioxidants, humectants, vitamins, and fatty acids, this shampoo will bring new life to hair of all kinds. After you've made it, don't hesitate to use it.

Ingredients:

1 tablespoon organic raw honey

2 tablespoons warm water

½ cup coconut oil

½ cup Flaxseed Gel for Hair (see page 122)

1 dash avocado oil

¼ cup liquid castile soap or True Liquid Castile Soap (see page 41)

10 drops rosemary essential oil

1   In a mixing bowl or pot, mix the honey and water.

2   Add the rest of the ingredients and stir to combine thoroughly.

3   Store sealed in a clean 12 OZ. shampoo bottle or jar in the fridge (so the Flaxseed Gel doesn't spoil) and use within 2 weeks.

Orange Peel Powder Shampoo Bar

This bar is meant to be stored in the shower and used every other day or a couple of times a week. For those with longer hair, you'll want to really take your time to work it in.

Ingredients:

⅔ cup extra-virgin olive oil

⅔ cup virgin coconut oil, melted

⅔ cup grapeseed oil

¼ cup sodium hydroxide (NaOH) lye flakes

¾ cup distilled water

2 tablespoons Orange Peel Powder (see sidebar)

1   In a stainless steel or plastic bowl, mix the oils together.

2   Working safely (see page 36), in another bowl add the lye to the distilled water, and let it cool to about 100°F.

3   Gently and carefully pour the lye solution into the bowl with the oils and stir.

4   Pour in the Orange Peel Powder and stir.

5   Using a hand mixer on low, beat the soap mixture to a gummy, translucent goop.

6   Pour the soap mixture into your mold(s) of choice and allow it to set for 24 hours.

7   Remove the hardened soap from the mold(s), cut into bars to your preference, and set in a cool, dark place to cure for at least 1 month before using.

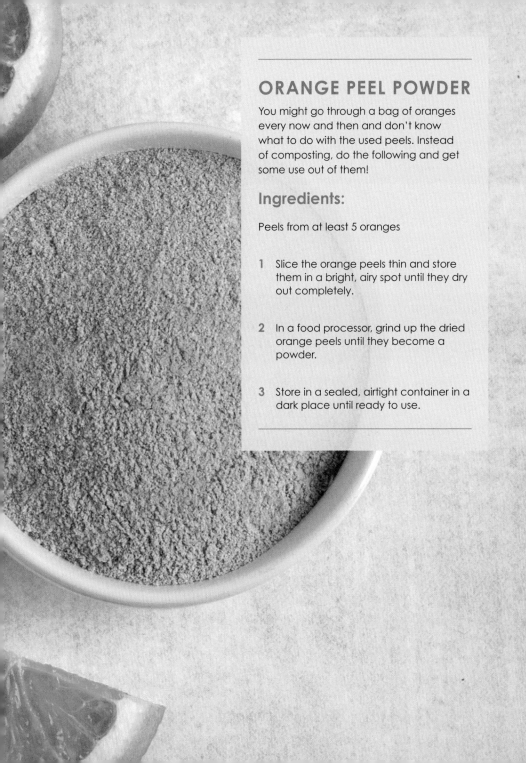

ORANGE PEEL POWDER

You might go through a bag of oranges every now and then and don't know what to do with the used peels. Instead of composting, do the following and get some use out of them!

Ingredients:

Peels from at least 5 oranges

1   Slice the orange peels thin and store them in a bright, airy spot until they dry out completely.

2   In a food processor, grind up the dried orange peels until they become a powder.

3   Store in a sealed, airtight container in a dark place until ready to use.

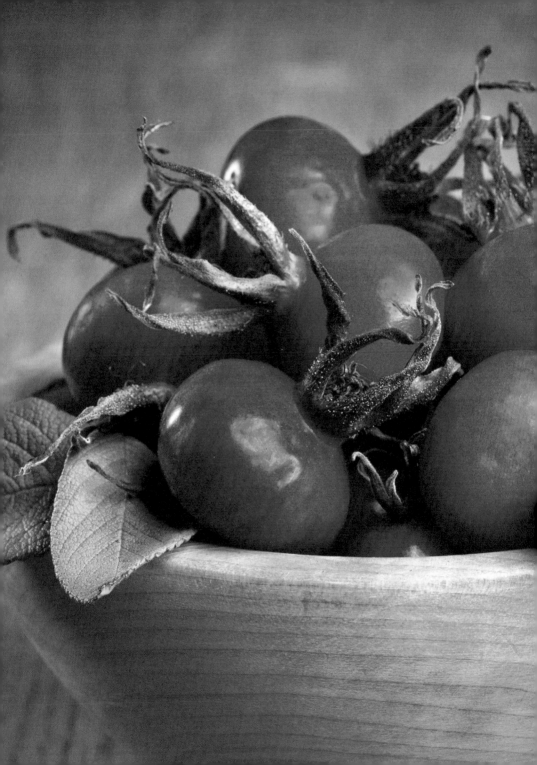

Rose Hip Hair Detangler

If you find that your hair simply isn't behaving or that it's too tough to brush through the tangles, then it's time for some extra love from Mother Nature. The oils in this recipe are packed with hair-juicing nutrition; rose hip seed oil is especially good for thick, textured hair, but feel free to substitute with any oil(s) you'd like.

Ingredients:

¼ cup coconut oil, melted

¼ cup extra-virgin olive oil

½ cup distilled water

20 drops rose hip seed oil

1   In a clean 8 OZ. spray bottle, add the ingredients and gently shake to combine.

2   Spray your hair liberally, working the detangler down to your roots, then brush.

Peppermint & Apple Cider Vinegar Conditioning Rinse

This light, watery conditioner will brighten and soften any type of hair, while giving your scalp a stimulating cleanse. If you don't like the pop of peppermint oil, substitute with another essential oil of your preference.

Ingredients:

5 tablespoons apple cider vinegar with the "Mother"

1¼ cups distilled water

20 drops peppermint essential oil

1   In a spray bottle or 12 OZ. reusable shampoo bottle, mix the ingredients together in order and gently shake to combine.

2   Apply once or twice a week, massaging it into your hair, and allow it to sit for about 5 minutes before rinsing thoroughly.

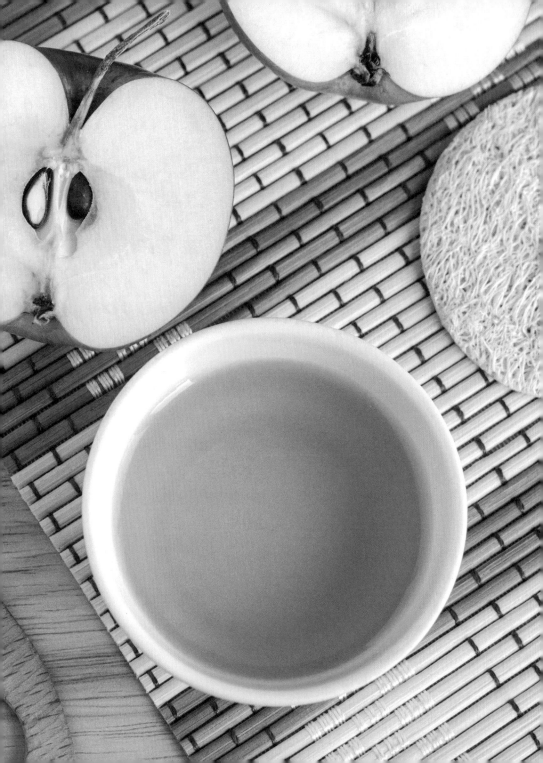

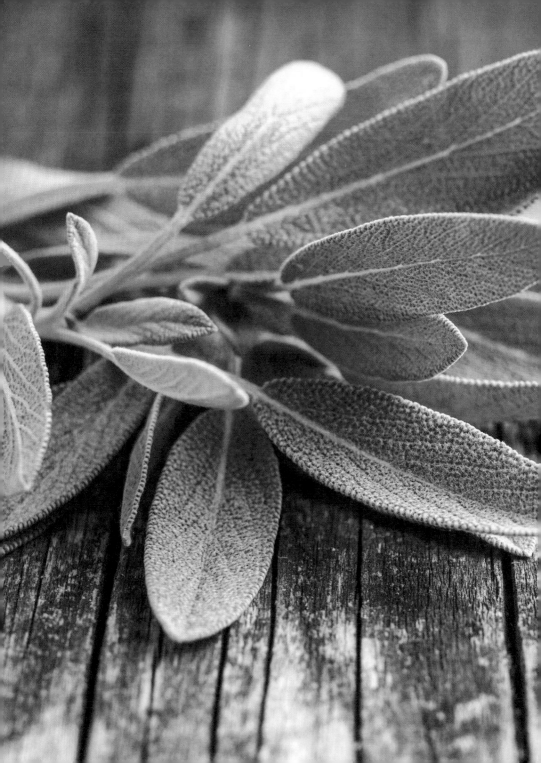

Sage Frizz-Control Hairspray

On those inevitable bad hair days or those days where the humidity is wreaking havoc on your hairdo, get a quick hit of this frizz-control spray. If you're not into the woodsy, herbal aroma of sage, try a classic scent like lavender or a brighter scent like lemon or grapefruit.

Ingredients:

7 OZ. distilled water

2 tablespoons grapeseed oil

10 to 15 drops sage essential oil

1 In an 8 OZ. spray bottle, add the ingredients and shake gently until combined.

2 Spray over your hair and work in with your fingers.

Coffee Hair Dye

Knock back the grayness and bring a new sharpness to your overall look with this natural hair dye. It works on beards too. Experiment with different coffee roasts and flavors, or use spent grounds instead of fresh.

Ingredients:

½ cup super-strong coffee, freshly brewed

2 tablespoons freshly ground coffee beans

1 cup Peppermint & Apple Cider Vinegar Conditioning Rinse (see page 130)

1   Brew some coffee. While you wait for the coffee to cool, wash your hair. Do not dry it completely.

2   Add the ground coffee beans to the ½ cup of brewed coffee.

3   In a jar, add the coffee mixture to the Peppermint & Apple Cider Vinegar Conditioning Rinse.

4   Using both a brush or comb and your hands, work the dye into your hair, down to the roots, and leave it in for at least an hour.

5   Rinse completely.

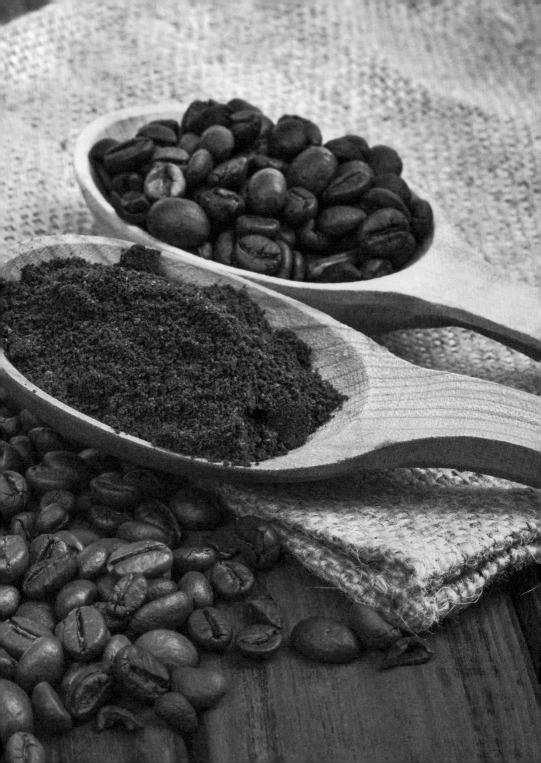

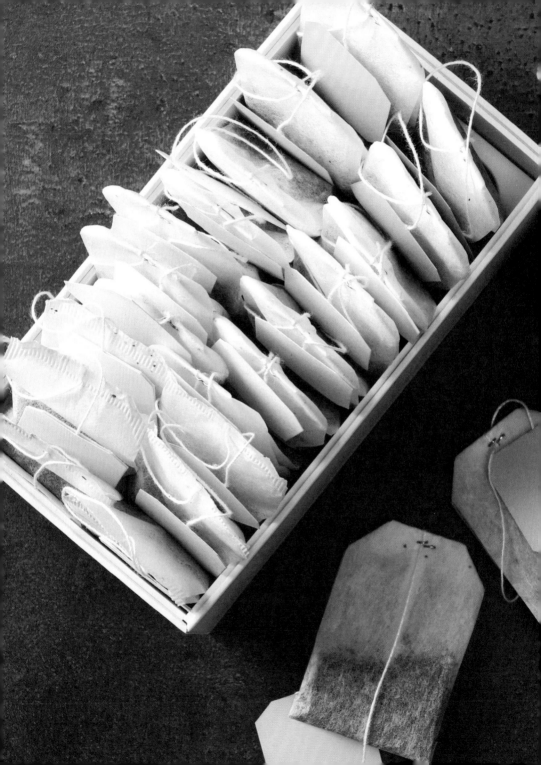

Green & Black Tea Rinse for Hair

This mix of teas—black for dying hair darker and green for stimulating growth—will be a good addition to your hair-care routine. Once a week, brew this recipe and let it work its magic.

Ingredients:

2 cups water

2 bags green tea

2 to 4 bags black tea

1 stem fresh oregano or rosemary

1   Boil the water, then add the tea bags and herbs and remove from heat. Allow the tea to steep for at least half an hour, or until cooled to room temperature.

2   Pour the tea mix (minus the herbs) into an 8 OZ. spray bottle.

3   After you've washed your hair and dried it, spray the tea rinse liberally all over your hair and work it in with your fingers.

4   Let it sit for an hour (you can wear a shower cap to keep your hair from drying too quickly), then rinse out with water.

Cedarwood Beard Oil

A beard (and the face underneath it) can benefit from a little TLC. This recipe will give a beard a rich, well-maintained look. You can substitute any essential oil or combination of oils for the cedarwood.

Ingredients:

1 tablespoon argan oil

½ tablespoon jojoba oil

½ tablespoon sweet almond oil

10 drops cedarwood essential oil

1   Combine all of the ingredients in a reusable stopper bottle and shake well.

2   Drop the oil onto your palm, apply it to the beard, and massage all the way down into the skin with your fingertips.

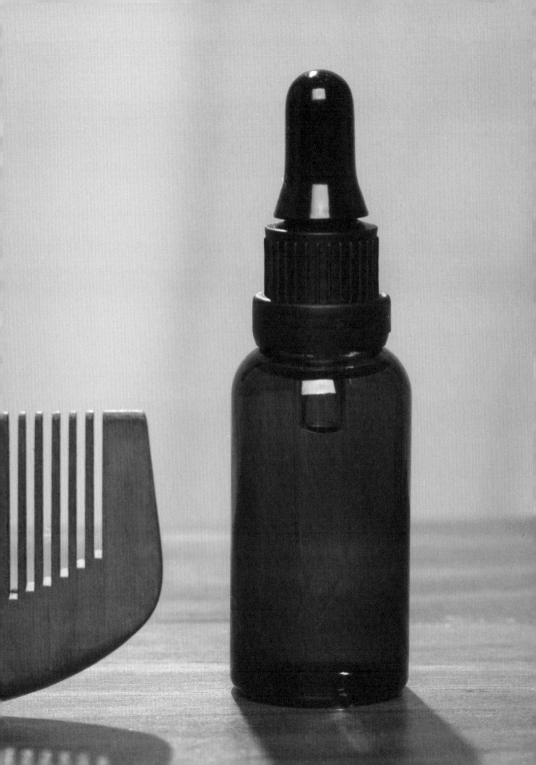

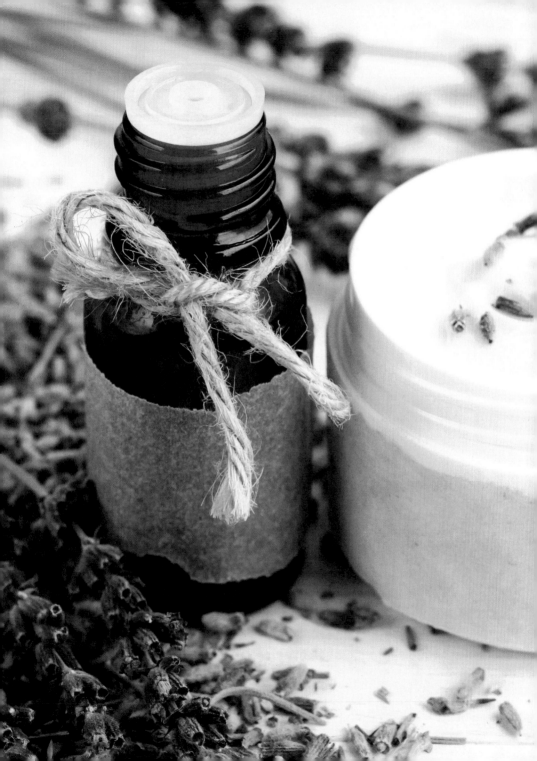

Sandalwood-Lavender Face Moisturizer Cream

Use this moisturizer daily after showering, and you can be assured that you're protecting your face with the best of the best. If you use this recipe frequently, get in the habit of tweaking an ingredient every time you make it—cocoa butter in place of shea butter, for example, or grapeseed oil instead of olive oil—until you find exactly what combination works best on your skin.

Ingredients:

½ cup shea butter

1 tablespoon jojoba oil

1 tablespoon organic extra-virgin olive oil

5 drops lavender essential oil

5 drops sandalwood essential oil

1   Set up your double boiler (see page 21) over low heat.

2   Add the shea butter, jojoba oil, and extra-virgin olive oil. As soon as they melt, remove from heat and stir to combine.

3   Add the essential oils and stir.

4   Pour into a 6 OZ. jar or tin and seal. Store in a cool place until ready to use.

Matcha-Honey Face Mask

In addition to matcha's antiaging powers, the honey moisturizes and shrinks pores, and the clays absorb any dirt or impurities. When you know you're due for some luxury, include this in your skin-care routine.

Ingredients:

½ teaspoon matcha

2 teaspoons kaolin clay

1 teaspoon bentonite clay

¼ teaspoon grapeseed oil

½ teaspoon honey, warmed

2 teaspoons distilled water

1 Mix the dry ingredients together in a bowl.

2 While stirring with a wooden spoon, add the wet ingredients. Stir until the mixture reaches a thick, paste-like consistency.

3 Use your fingers or a face mask brush to apply the mask material to your face.

4 Before the mask dries completely—about 10 minutes—remove the mask with a warm, wet towel. Moisturize immediately after use.

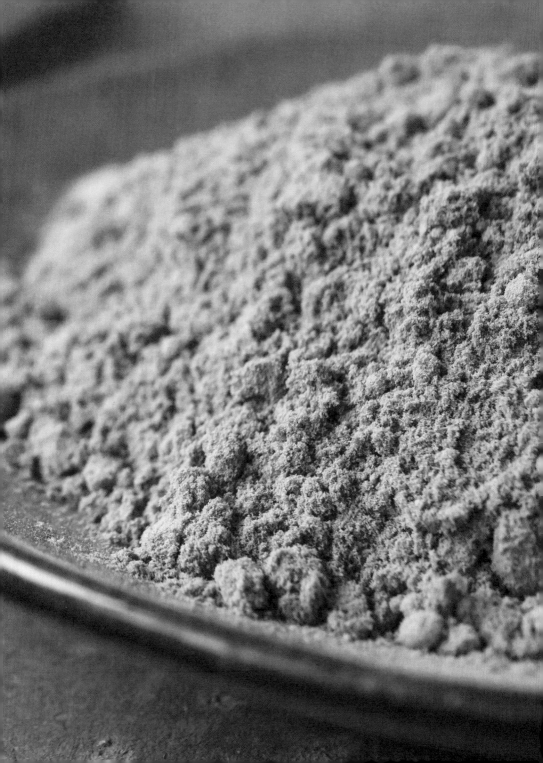

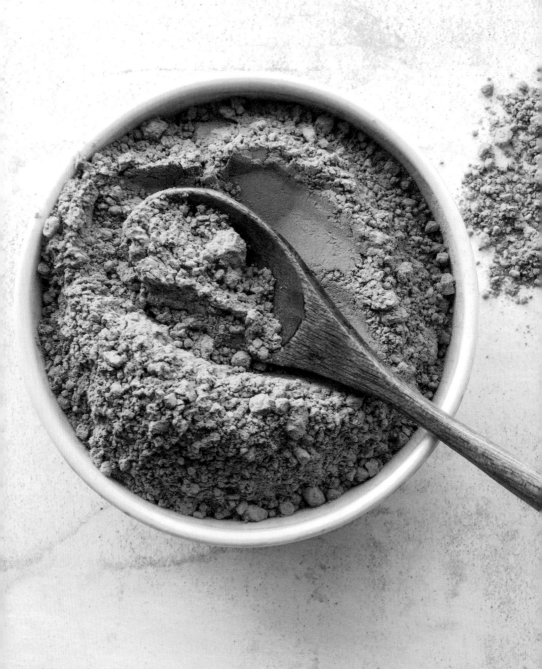

Antiaging Matcha–Kaolin Clay Face Mask

Roll back the years and smooth out any wrinkles with this antioxidant-rich matcha face mask. Kaolin clay is the gentlest clay out there, and it will leave your face feeling irresistibly smooth.

Ingredients:

2 tablespoons kaolin clay

1 teaspoon matcha powder

4 tablespoons distilled water

1   In a bowl, mix all of the ingredients together into a creamy paste.

2   Store in a sealed 2 OZ. jar until ready for use.

3   To use, apply to the face with a face mask brush or your fingers and allow it to set for 5 to 10 minutes. Using a warm, wet towel, remove the mask before it dries, and moisturize immediately afterward.

Coffee-Vanilla Face Scrub

Store this face scrub in a small, sealed glass jar. Every few days, or whenever you need a pick-me-up, you can use this rich, aromatic scrub to exfoliate.

Ingredients:

½ cup granulated sugar

¼ cup coffee grounds

¼ cup coconut oil, melted

1 teaspoon vanilla extract

1   Mix the sugar and coffee grounds together in a wooden, metal, or glass bowl. Meanwhile, gently melt the coconut oil by microwaving it in 10-second intervals, stirring between intervals.

2   Stir in the coconut oil and vanilla extract until it reaches a clumpy, paste-like consistency.

3   When cool, use your fingers to apply in small amounts to your face and neck, and massage the scrub onto your skin. Rinse the scrub off when finished.

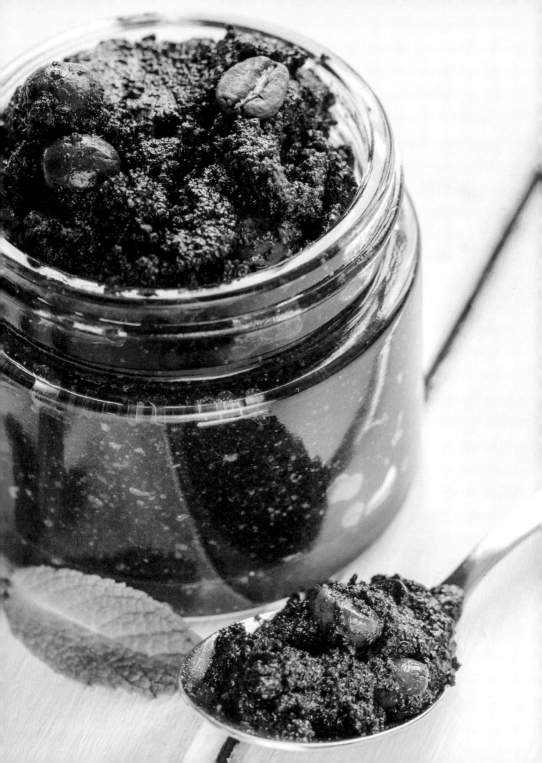

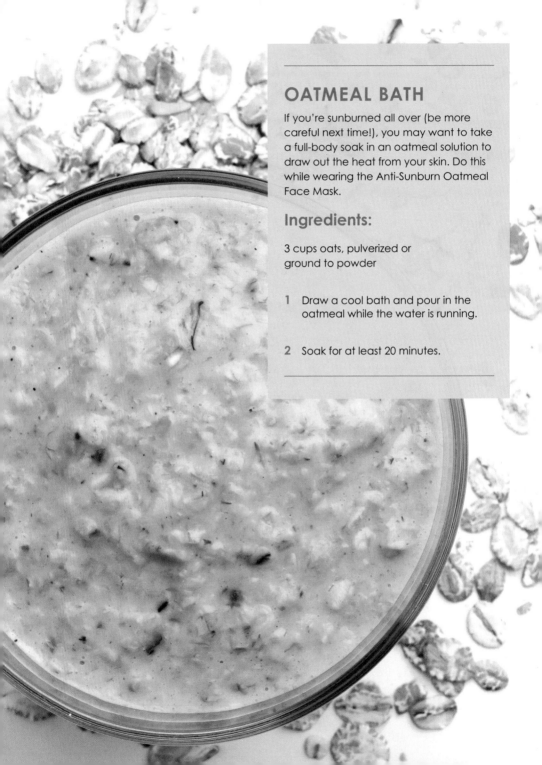

OATMEAL BATH

If you're sunburned all over (be more careful next time!), you may want to take a full-body soak in an oatmeal solution to draw out the heat from your skin. Do this while wearing the Anti-Sunburn Oatmeal Face Mask.

Ingredients:

3 cups oats, pulverized or ground to powder

1   Draw a cool bath and pour in the oatmeal while the water is running.

2   Soak for at least 20 minutes.

Anti-Sunburn Oatmeal Face Mask

When you wind up outside on a sunny day and you've left your sunscreen at home, within minutes the sun can take a toll on your face. Not to worry: if you have this waiting for you in the fridge at home, you can counteract the damage.

Ingredients:

½ cup distilled water

2 bags chamomile tea

½ cup oats, pulverized or ground to powder

1 teaspoon organic honey

1   Boil the distilled water and steep the tea bags to make a concentrated tea.

2   In a bowl, slowly mix the oats, tea, and honey while stirring.

3   If the paste is too dry, add more distilled water.

4   Refrigerate until cool before applying. Once the mask has done its job, remove it with a cool, wet washcloth before it dries.

Apple Cider Vinegar Face Toner

Use this anytime throughout the day when you want to get your glow back. This toner will also help combat skin issues. Apply with reusable cotton rounds.

Ingredients:

¾ cup distilled water

3 tablespoons apple cider vinegar with the "Mother"

1 tablespoon grapeseed oil

10 drops lavender essential oil

1   In an 8 OZ. jar or bottle, add all of the ingredients and shake gently to combine.

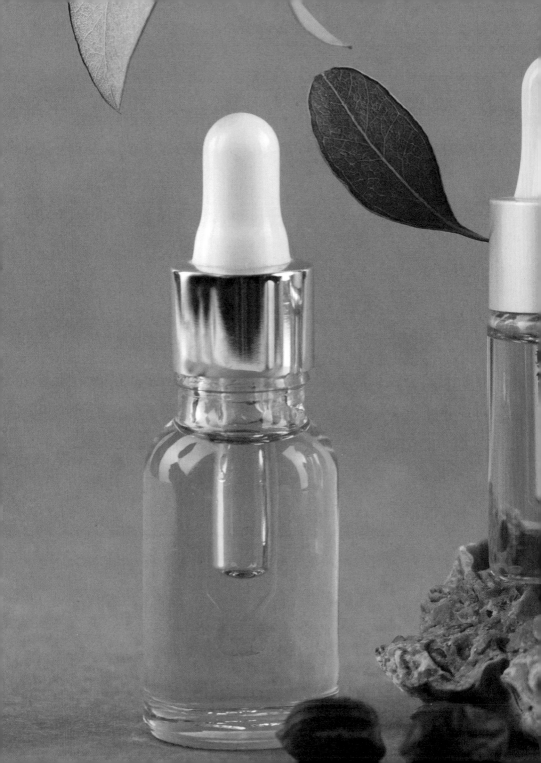

After-Shower Wake-Up Spritz

This is the perfect addition to your morning routine. After you've showered and toweled off, give yourself the jojoba glow before taking on the world with this easy-to-make spray.

Ingredients:

1½ cups distilled water

¼ cup jojoba oil

10 drops eucalyptus essential oil

1   In a clean 16 OZ. spray bottle, add the distilled water and then the essential oils.

2   Shake gently to mix, and then shake again before each use.

3   Spray over clean skin and hair and, using your fingers, work the spray in, scalp included.

Calendula Oil

If you aren't already, you should be growing a pot or two of *Calendula officinalis*—aka pot marigolds or English/Scotch marigolds—a showy orange or yellow flower that looks at home in any flower garden. It is also known for its medicinal properties. This oil is your go-to for skin ailments and irritations of all kinds.

Ingredients:

4 to 6 tablespoons dried calendula flower heads or petals

½ cup jojoba oil

1   Pour the calendula into the jar, then fill the jar with the jojoba oil.

2   Seal the jar and place it in a warm, sunny location for a month to allow the petals to completely infuse the oil.

3   Strain the oil infusion into a separate clean jar or glass bottle and store at room temperature when not in use.

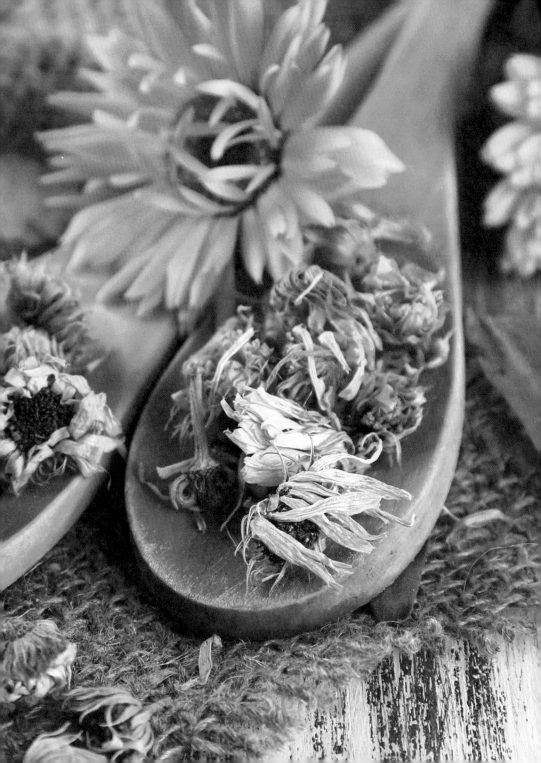

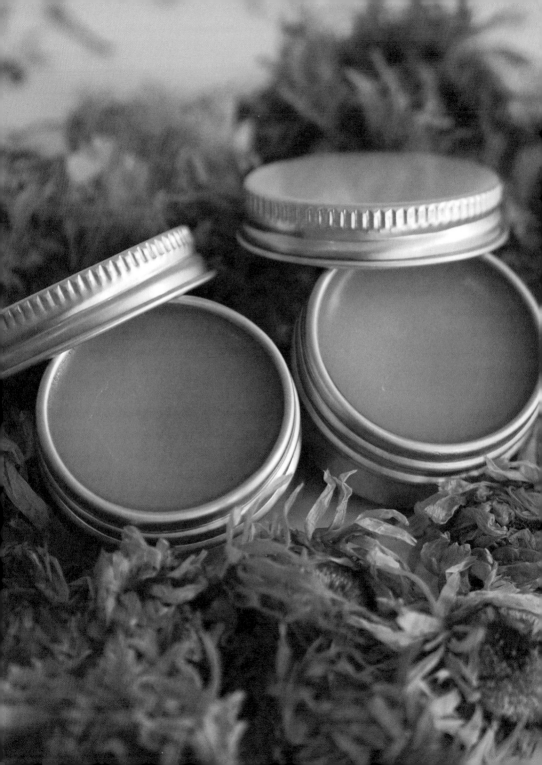

Rosemary-Calendula Skin Salve

This gentle skin salve can be used on any skin irritation: bug bites, sunburns, boo-boos, diaper rash, poison ivy rash, and scalds. If you prefer a cooler-scented salve, use lavender oil instead of rosemary.

Ingredients:

½ cup Calendula Oil (see page 154)

2 tablespoons beeswax pellets

5 to 10 drops rosemary essential oil

1 Set up your double boiler (see page 21) over low heat.

2 Add the ingredients to the double boiler in order and stir slowly to melt the beeswax.

3 Once the beeswax is completely melted, stir to combine and quickly remove from heat.

4 Carefully pour the salve mixture into your container(s) of choice. Set aside, lid(s) off, to cool completely and solidify before using or storing.

Calendula-Frankincense Lotion Bars

Since shea butter has a melting point of about 90°F, these bars will travel well. Whenever you feel that your skin could use an extra dose of TLC—say, your feet after a day of hiking—hit it with this bar. Allow your body heat to melt the bar on extended contact. Compare this recipe with the Lavender Moisturizer Travel Bars on page 162.

Ingredients:

¼ cup beeswax pellets

¼ cup shea butter

¼ cup Calendula Oil (see page 154)

10 to 15 drops frankincense essential oil

1   Set up your double boiler (see page 21) over low heat.

2   Add the beeswax and shea butter. Stir until they are melted and combined, then immediately remove from heat.

3   Add the Calendula Oil and frankincense essential oil and stir to combine.

4   Pour the mixture into your bar mold(s) of choice and let it cool for a few hours.

5   Remove from the mold(s) and cut into bars.

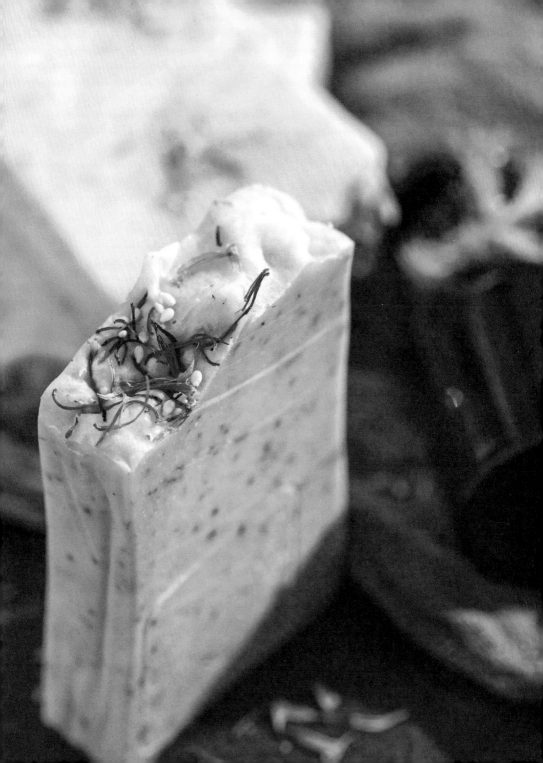

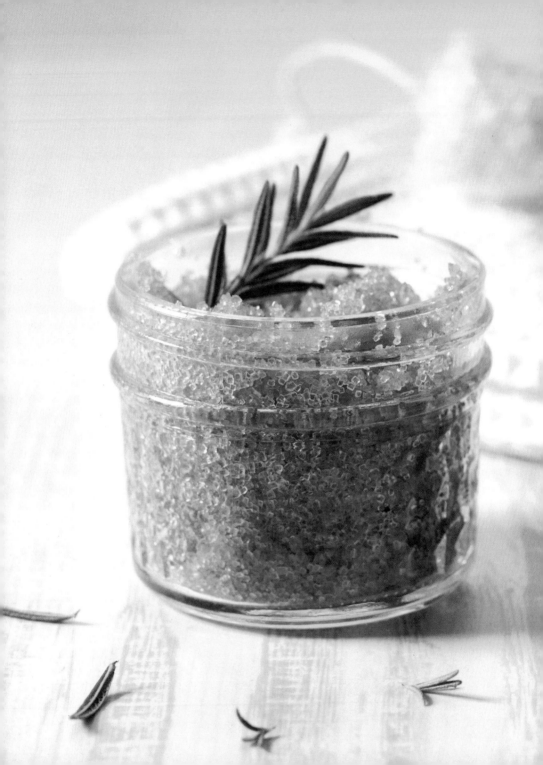

Bergamot & Brown Sugar Antiaging Sugar Scrub

After a bath or shower, massage this exfoliating scrub over your face and body. This recipe is best if used up within a month or two—and your skin will show the difference!

Ingredients:

1 cup organic brown sugar

3 tablespoons apricot kernel oil

5 to 10 drops bergamot essential oil

1   In a bowl, add the sugar and slowly combine with the apricot kernel oil while stirring.

2   Add the essential oil and stir.

3   Store in a sealed 10 OZ. jar until ready to use.

Lavender Moisturizer Travel Bars

You'll need a mold for this recipe—a cookie pan will do. These moisturizer bars are solid, and therefore good to take on the road, but on contact with your skin they will melt and give your skin a luxuriant touch-up. Compare this recipe with the Calendula-Frankincense Lotion Bars on page 158.

Ingredients:

5 tablespoons coconut oil

5 tablespoons shea butter

5½ tablespoons beeswax pellets

5 to 10 drops lavender essential oil, or preferred oil

1   Combine the coconut oil, shea butter, and beeswax in a microwave-safe bowl or in a double boiler (see page 21) and melt them together, stirring gently.

2   Add the essential oil.

3   Pour the heated mixture into your molds of choice and allow it to cool completely.

4   Store in containers or in burlap cloth in the fridge when not in use.

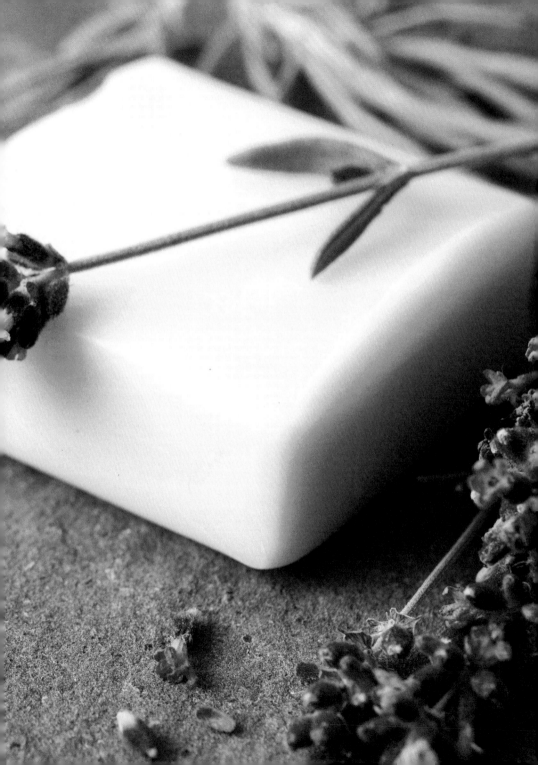

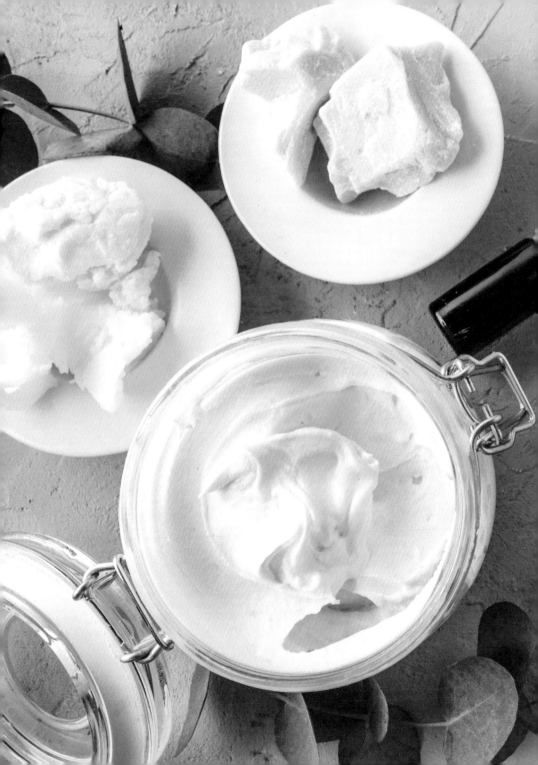

Floral Body Butter

Massage this body butter into your skin (or your hair) whenever you feel like it. The carrier oils will revitalize thirsty, dry skin, and the vibrant aromas will awaken the senses. Note that the whipping process in step 5 will be easier with an electric hand mixer, but a hand whisk will do the job too.

Ingredients:

½ cup coconut oil

½ cup shea butter

¼ cup sweet almond oil

10 drops jasmine essential oil

10 drops lavender essential oil

Lavender stems, flowers, and petals (optional)

1   Set up your double boiler (see page 21) over low heat.

2   Add the coconut oil and shea butter and stir gently until melted.

3   Add the sweet almond oil and remove from heat, continuing to stir until combined. Allow it to cool.

4   Add the essential oils, stir, and refrigerate for 1 hour.

5   Whip the mixture to a buttery, fluffy consistency and transfer to a 10 OZ. jar. Add the lavender, if desired, and seal, storing in a cool place until ready to use.

Meditative Bath Soak

The woody, sweet scent of the frankincense, plus the deep calm that comes from the lavender, will bring peace and relief to the senses. Meanwhile, the apple cider vinegar will exfoliate and detoxify your skin and have you emerge glowing.

Ingredients:

1½ cups apple cider vinegar with the "Mother"

1 cup Epsom salts

5 to 10 drops frankincense essential oil

5 to 10 drops lavender essential oil

1   While the hot bath is running, dump the apple cider vinegar and then the salts under the stream and mix them in.

2   Add the essential oils and allow the tub to fill to your preferred level. Enter the bath when ready.

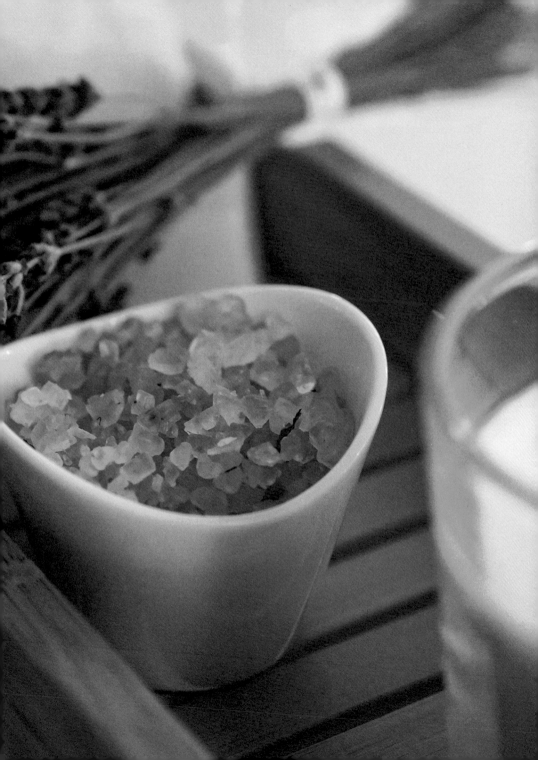

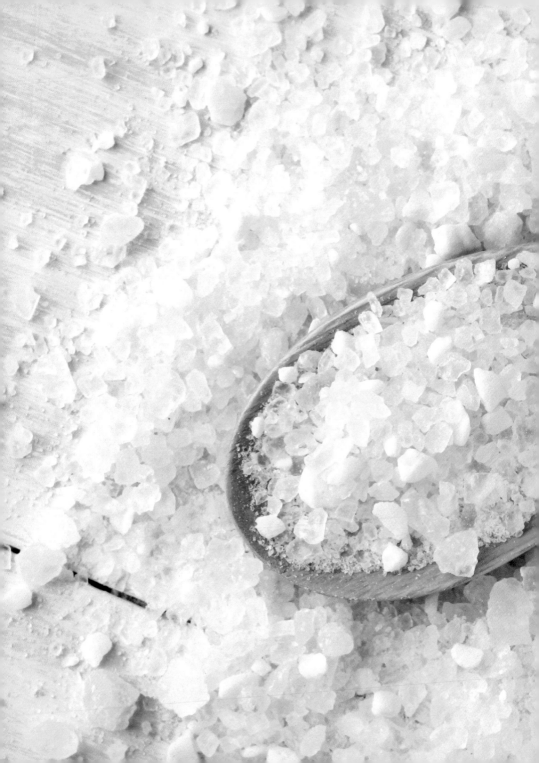

Chamomile-Sandalwood Bath Salts

If you've had an active day and you want to really relax before bed, soaking in a tub with this mix will soothe your aches and pains and help you decompress. The Epsom salts and baking soda will exfoliate tired feet in short order.

Ingredients:

2 cups Epsom salts

½ cup baking soda

½ cup fine sea salt

10 drops sandalwood essential oil

5 bags chamomile tea

1   Mix the Epsom salts, baking soda, and sea salt together in a large, clean jar.

2   Add the essential oil and stir to mix. Seal the jar and store in a cool, dry place until ready to use.

3   To use, run a hot bath. While the bath is filling, tip the jar into the running stream. Add the tea bags and allow the tub to fill to your preferred level. Enter the bath when ready.

Basic Foot Soak

To remove dead skin and soften calluses, there's no easier way than an exfoliating foot soak. This one can be whipped up in no time at all.

Ingredients:

½ cup baking soda

2 gallons hot or warm water

1   Mix the ingredients in a basin or foot spa.

2   Relax and soak for about 20 minutes, then moisturize your feet after.

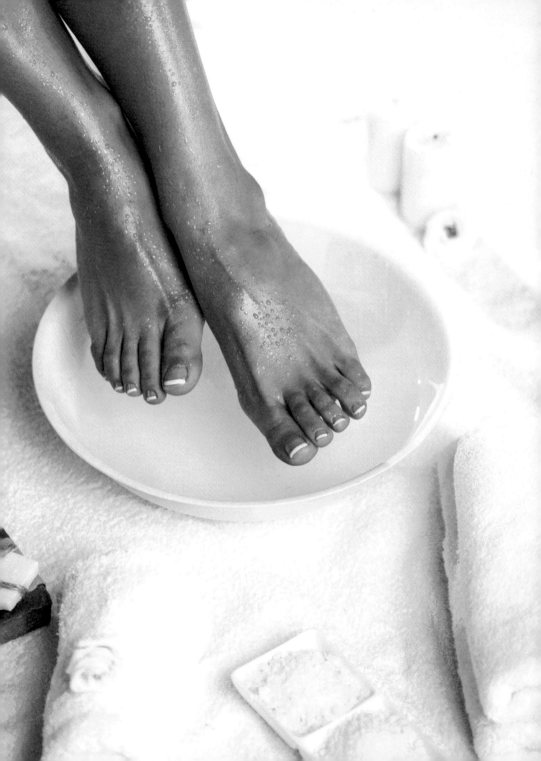

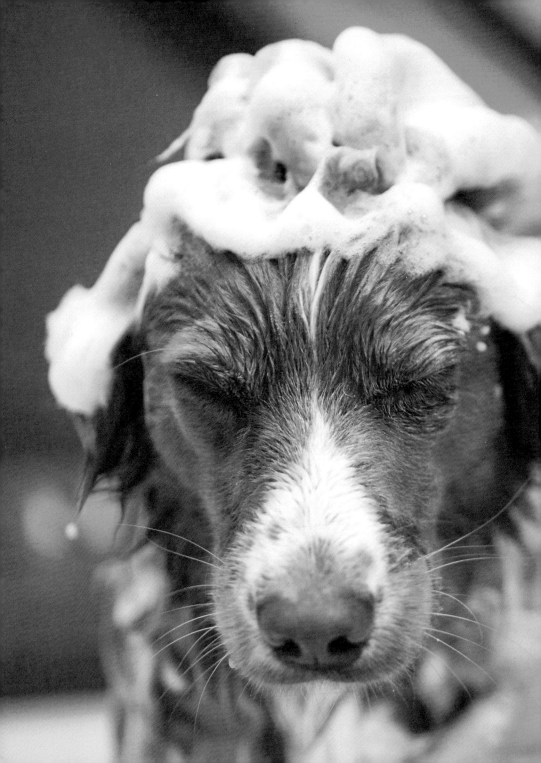

Easy-on-the-Fur Dog Shampoo

If your furry friend's coat isn't at its best, it's probably time for a dog bath. This recipe will have your dog smelling great and feeling refreshed in no time. Just avoid lathering too closely to the eyes, nose, and mouth.

Ingredients:

1 cup liquid castile soap or True Liquid Castile Soap (see page 41)

6 tablespoons baking soda

8 cups water

1 to 2 drops preferred essential oil

1   Add the ingredients to a jug or large bottle.

2   Cap the container and shake moderately until the mixture is uniformly white.

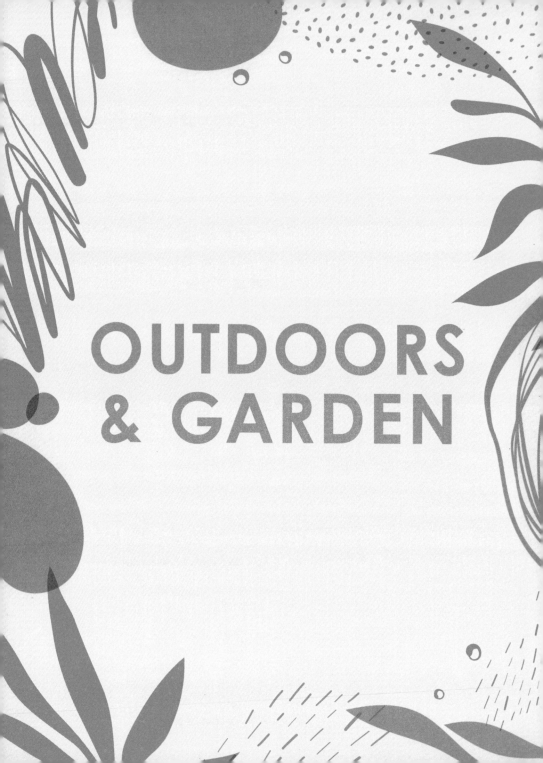

OUTDOORS
& GARDEN

Nobody wants to spray their plants with the harmful toxins found in store-bought insecticides and pesticides. These recipes will help you eliminate harmful critters and create healthful fertilizers for your home garden. Make sure you target the right insects, and avoid killing beneficial bugs and plants!

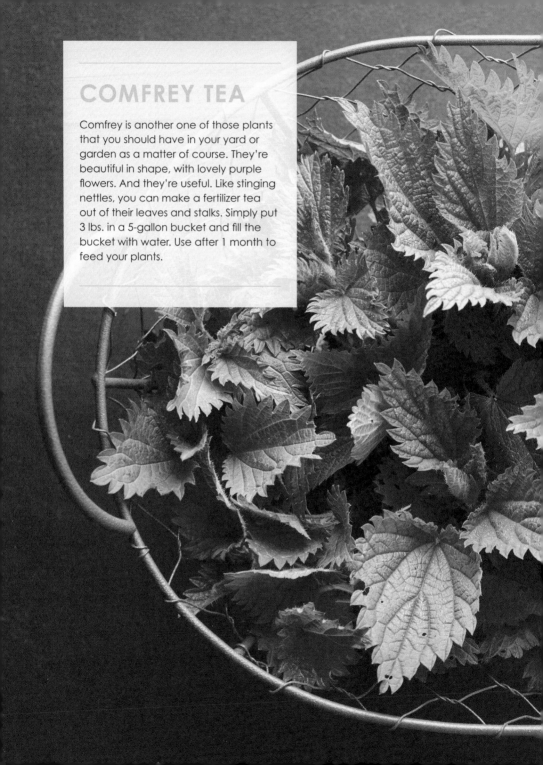

COMFREY TEA

Comfrey is another one of those plants that you should have in your yard or garden as a matter of course. They're beautiful in shape, with lovely purple flowers. And they're useful. Like stinging nettles, you can make a fertilizer tea out of their leaves and stalks. Simply put 3 lbs. in a 5-gallon bucket and fill the bucket with water. Use after 1 month to feed your plants.

Stinging Nettle Plant Food

Stinging nettle (*Urtica dioica*), aka common nettle or burn hazel, grows prolifically in the wild and makes for a memorable encounter if your skin happens to brush against its needles. However, it also can be used to make a potent organic fertilizer. Here's an opportunity to indulge your inner forager. Just remember your gloves!

Ingredients:

2 lbs. nettles

5 gallons water

1   After carefully harvesting the nettles, place the plants in a 5-gallon bucket and fill the bucket with water. If you have a rain barrel, use the water from that. If you prefer, you can reuse an old onion bag to contain the nettles for easy removal later.

2   After two weeks, remove the nettles. The infused water can be used to feed plants in your garden or in your house.

Garden Herbicide

If you have a problem with weeds, this simple recipe will help you eradicate them. If it's a large, woody weed, a shrub, or even a small tree, first hack it back as much as you can, and then soak the exposed inner wood. You'll probably need to repeat this process more than once.

Ingredients:

4 heaping tablespoons salt

3 cups distilled white vinegar

5 OZ. Citrus Punch Hand-Wash & Dish Soap (see page 71)

1   In a 32 OZ. spray bottle, add the salt, then the vinegar, and shake to dissolve the salt.

2   Add the dish soap and shake gently to mix. Store out of reach of children until ready to use.

3   Shake before use, then spray the weeds liberally on a windless, sunny day. Repeat as necessary until the weeds are killed, being careful to avoid accidentally spraying nearby plants.

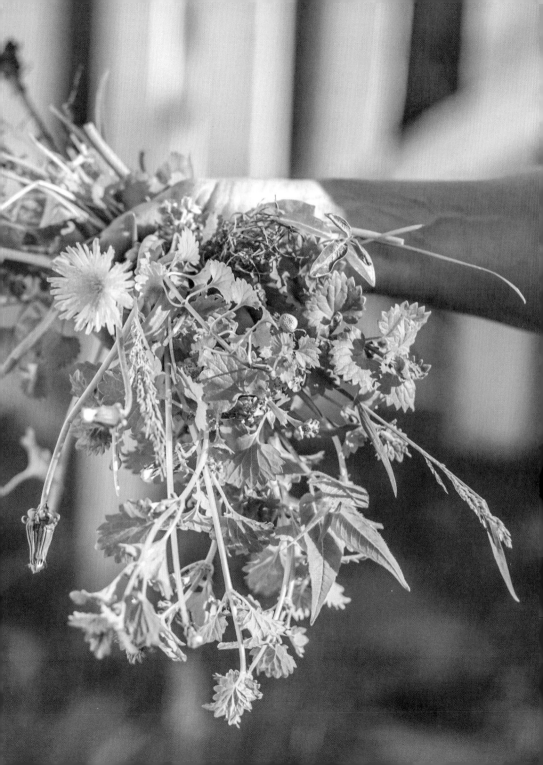

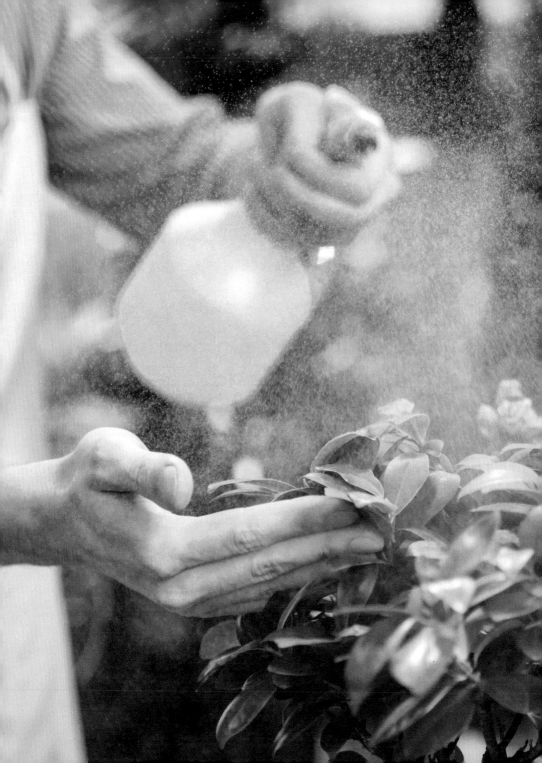

Garden Insecticide

In a perfect world, your garden's "good" bugs would easily handle its "bad" bugs on their own, without any help from you. However, as that's not usually the case, if you spot an infestation of squash bugs, Colorado potato beetles, flea beetles, or any other notorious garden pest, give them a few blasts with this spray daily for about a week to bring the balance back. Just be sure to identify the bugs first—the last thing you want to do is spray the good guys.

Ingredients:

4 cups distilled water

1 tablespoon liquid castile soap or True Liquid Castile Soap (see page 41)

1 tablespoon neem essential oil

1   In a 32 OZ. spray bottle that you dedicate to this recipe, combine all of the ingredients.

2   Shake gently to mix, and then shake again before each use.

3   Spray onto the offending garden pests. The spray works by suffocating the bugs, so aim to really soak them.

Mosquito Repellent Skin Spray

With a loaded spray bottle in hand, you can reclaim your backyard during the summer mosquito months while avoiding the harmful chemicals of off-the-shelf insect repellents. Bugs dislike citronella and peppermint scents, and the jojoba oil will help the spray go smoothly on your skin.

Ingredients:

1¾ cups distilled water

20 drops citronella essential oil

20 drops peppermint essential oil

1 tablespoon jojoba oil

1 In a clean 16 OZ. spray bottle that you dedicate to this recipe, add the distilled water and then the rest of the ingredients.

2 Shake gently to mix, and then shake again before each use.

3 Spray onto your exposed skin sparingly, as needed. Reapply every few hours.

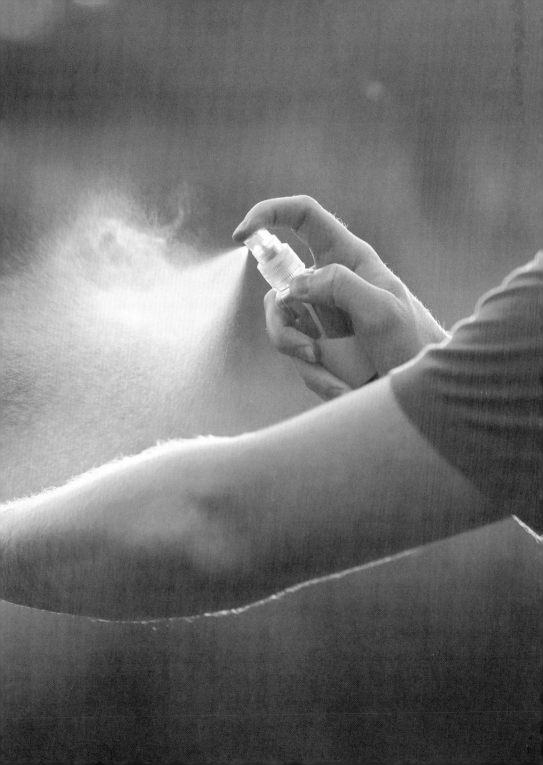

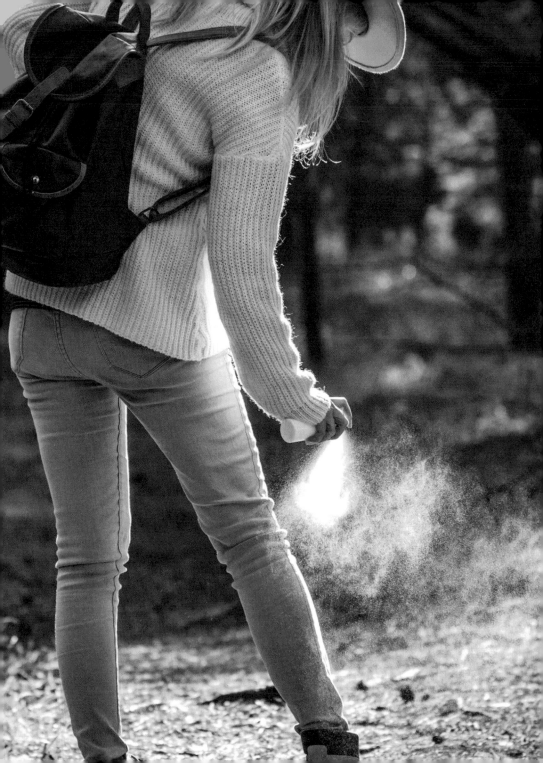

Tick Repellent Spray

Take no chances with ticks: always wear long pants if you're hiking or camping in areas where ticks are known to be. Spray this repellant frequently, especially around your feet, ankles, and lower legs. This recipe can do double duty against mosquitoes and flies as well.

Ingredients:

1 cup distilled water

60 drops geranium essential oil

60 drops cedarwood essential oil

40 drops peppermint essential oil

1 In an 8 OZ. spray bottle, add the distilled water then the essential oils and shake gently to combine.

2 Store in a cool, dark place out of reach of children until ready to use. Shake before each use and spray liberally.

METRIC CONVERSION CHART

U.S. Measurement	Approximate Metric Liquid Measurement	Approximate Metric Dry Measurement
1 teaspoon	5 ml	5 g
1 tablespoon or ½ ounce	15 ml	14 g
1 ounce or ⅛ cup	30 ml	29 g
¼ cup or 2 ounces	60 ml	57 g
⅓ cup	80 ml	76 g
½ cup or 4 ounces	120 ml	113 g
⅔ cup	160 ml	151 g
¾ cup or 6 ounces	180 ml	170 g
1 cup or 8 ounces or ½ pint	240 ml	227 g
1½ cups or 12 ounces	350 ml	340 g
2 cups or 1 pint or 16 ounces	475 ml	454 g
3 cups or 1½ pints	700 ml	680 g
4 cups or 2 pints or 1 quart	950 ml	908 g

INDEX

ABOUT CIDER MILL PRESS
BOOK PUBLISHERS

Good ideas ripen with time. From seed to harvest, Cider Mill Press brings fine reading, information, and entertainment together between the covers of its creatively crafted books. Our Cider Mill bears fruit twice a year, publishing a new crop of titles each spring and fall.

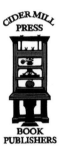

"Where Good Books Are Ready for Press"

Visit us online at
cidermillpress.com

or write to us at
501 Nelson Place
Nashville, Tennessee 37214

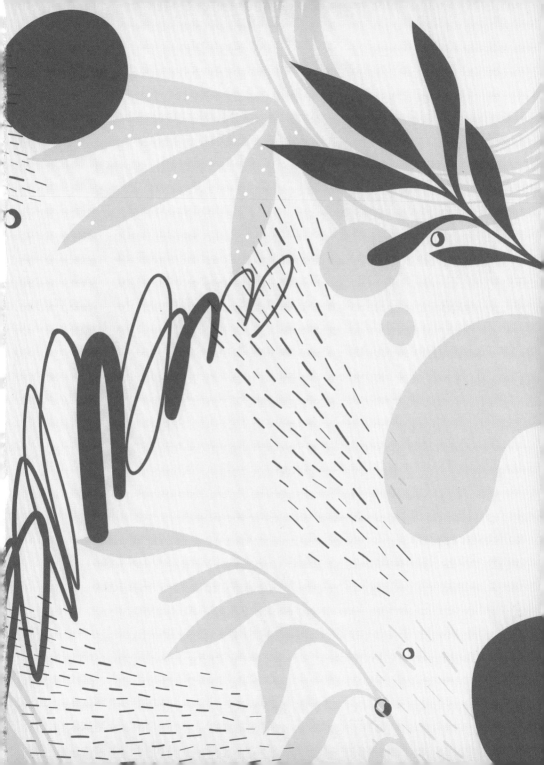

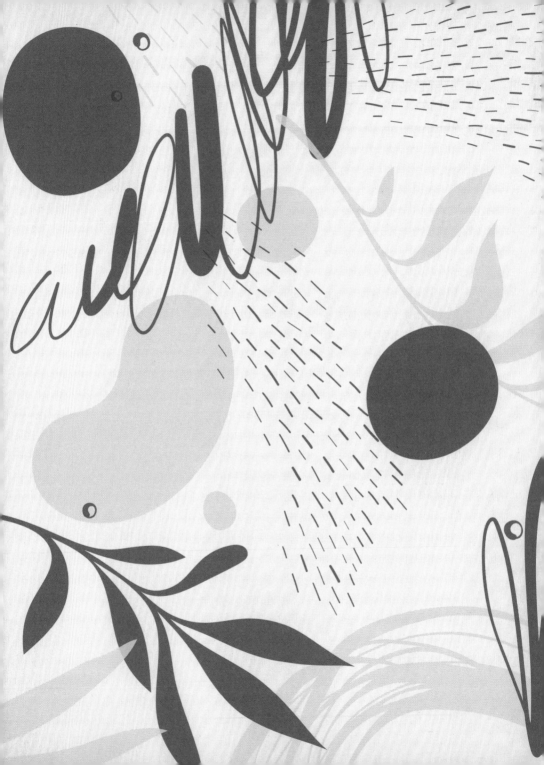